Weighty Problems

Weighty Problems

Embodied Inequality at a Children's Weight Loss Camp

LAURA BACKSTROM

Rutgers University Press

New Brunswick, Camden, and Newark, New Jersey, and London

Library of Congress Cataloging-in-Publication Data

Names: Backstrom, Laura, author.
Title: Weighty problems : embodied inequality at a children's weight loss camp /
    Laura Backstrom.
Description: New Brunswick : Rutgers University Press, [2019] | Includes bibliographical
    references and index.
Identifiers: LCCN 2018022089 | ISBN 9780813599120 (cloth) | ISBN 9780813599113
    (paperback)
Subjects: LCSH: Obesity in children—Psychological aspects. | Weight loss—Psychological
    aspects. | Body image in children.
Classification: LCC RJ399.C6 B33 2019 | DDC 618.92/398—dc23
LC record available at https://lccn.loc.gov/2018022089

A British Cataloging-in-Publication record for this book is available from the British Library.

♾ The paper used in this publication meets the requirements of the American National
Standard for Information Sciences—Permanence of Paper for Printed Library Materials,
ANSI Z39.48-1992.

www.rutgersuniversitypress.org

Manufactured in the United States of America

Contents

Weighty Problems

1

Embodied Inequality, Childhood Obesity, and the "Problem Child"

The children awake in their bunk beds to the squeals of campers chasing each other to communal bathrooms. Near their cabin is a fire pit with the charred remains of last night's campfire where they had spent the evening hours singing songs and impersonating the counselors. Down the dirt path about a half mile is a lake with a dock and large inflatables where the children will splash around in the still chilly water later that day. Spread across the 600 wooded acres of the campground, there are arts and crafts buildings, a ropes course, a dining hall, open fields, basketball and tennis courts, and two pools. It is the quintessential summer camp, a rite of passage for thousands of American children.

Yet these campers differ in one key way: they came to Camp Odyssey to lose weight. Unlike other summer camps, Odyssey campers are given a pretest that includes measures of their height, weight, body mass index (BMI), body fat percentage, blood pressure, and the circumference of five parts of their body as well as fitness tests. Camp Odyssey is a weight loss camp located in a midwestern town that draws thousands of visitors to its waterparks and tourist attractions during the summer. A few miles from the souvenir shops and restaurants of downtown is Camp Jay, a large campground that is operated by the Jewish Community Center (JCC) of a nearby city. Camp Odyssey is embedded in this larger camp, but it is not affiliated with the JCC. For the past decade, Fay and Steve, the married camp directors of Odyssey, have rented a small number of cabins for their twenty to forty participants and paid for the use of Camp Jay's facilities and dining services. Odyssey campers follow a separate program of activities and have little interaction with Jay campers.

On this June morning during the first week of camp, the campers change into T-shirts and athletic shorts, fill their water bottles, and head to the dining hall for breakfast. Hundreds of Camp Jay campers are already there. There are long tables at the front of the room filled with a buffet of breakfast items, including pastries, sugary cereals, tubs of peanut butter and jelly, and fresh fruit. The Odyssey campers sit at the four tables designated for them. A counselor brings over a sample plate to show the campers which foods they can eat from the buffet and the portion sizes they should take. The campers eat carefully portioned meals totaling about 1,800 calories per day.

Following breakfast, the campers go to Odyssey Time, which consists of three forty-five-minute rotations. One rotation, a weight loss information session, is called Education and is nearly always led by Fay, the camp codirector. The second rotation is Movement, a structured exercise class such as kickboxing, yoga, or dance. The third rotation can consist of a guest speaker on nutrition, a body image workshop, a self-defense class, or fitness tests. Campers stay at camp for two weeks or a month. For the first two weeks, campers are divided into three groups: older girls, younger girls, and boys. During the second two weeks, the number of campers is small enough that they are simply divided into two groups based on gender.

After Odyssey Time, the campers walk to the gym where they play dodgeball before going to lunch at the dining hall. After lunch, they change into their swimsuits and head to the pool, where the boys play an aggressive game of basketball in the shallow end while the girls play Marco Polo in the deep end. Still in their swimsuits, the campers walk to the lake where they have a snack of pita chips, vegetables, and hummus. At 5 P.M., they go back to their cabins to change for a cookout at the picnic grove. After they eat grilled chicken and vegetables, the counselors go around with face paint. In the evening, they have a social activity, such as karaoke, movie night, or a camp dance. On this particular night, they paint murals to decorate their cabin doors and invent cabin nicknames like "The Extreme Eight." By 8:30 P.M., the counselors usher them back to the cabins for showers and quiet time before lights out at 10 P.M.

In many ways, this June day was a typical day at a typical summer camp. In other ways, the campers were engaged in a program of bodily and self-change that was anything but ordinary. Although several weight loss camps have operated for decades, the growing acceptance of intensive weight management programs for children is directly linked to more recent concerns—even panic—about childhood obesity. As children are exposed to messages about weight control at earlier ages, antiobesity programs have become important sites of cultural meaning about body size. Thousands of children have attended one of the approximately two dozen summer weight loss camps in the United States.[1]

Many parents, teachers, and doctors believe that childhood obesity is a social problem that needs to be solved. Yet missing from debates over what caused the rise in childhood obesity and how to fix it are the children themselves. What is it like to grow up worried about your weight? How does weight affect children's relationships with their peers and families? How do children learn that their bodies are problems and that they should try to change the way they look? How does participating in a weight loss program affect a child's developing self-image? This book turns the spotlight on children's firsthand experiences and understandings of the cultural meanings surrounding body size and how they learn about embodied inequality.

Childhood Obesity as a Social Problem

In February 2010, Michelle Obama launched her national antiobesity campaign called Let's Move! The following May, the White House Task Force on Childhood Obesity released a 120-page report that provided the guiding standards for the Let's Move! program. In this report, the goal of the campaign was stated as long term: to lower the childhood obesity rate from 17 percent to 5 percent by 2030. While many initiatives arose over the past decade to address childhood obesity, Let's Move! garnered a great deal of media attention and became the most recognizable antiobesity campaign. In Fall 2011, a few months after the camp session ended, Michelle Obama gave a speech at the Partnership for Healthier America in which she said, "So when we're talking about getting kids running around and playing again, it is important to understand that this isn't just about fun and games. This isn't a joke. It's about their health. It's about their success in school. It's about our economy. It's about our national security."

For Mrs. Obama, childhood obesity signified cultural and institutional problems within society that threatened the nation's future. For the young people who attended Camp Odyssey, childhood obesity was more personal. They saw their weight as an added burden to the problems of growing up, and one that required enormous effort to resolve. The success of Let's Move! and the growing popularity of weight loss programs for children raise an important question about contemporary American culture: Why has children's body size become a central issue to so many people?

One answer to this question is based on observed changes in the population's body size. In the 1990s, health officials noted that BMI had risen among the American population since the 1970s.[2] The percentage of children aged 2 to 19 who are considered to be obese has more than tripled in the past thirty years to 17 percent.[3] Many government and medical studies viewed the increasing obesity rate as a public health crisis.[4] While childhood obesity trends reflect broader patterns of increasing obesity rates among adults, the rhetoric is amplified because children are involved. Many in the medical community, media, and government warn of health risks associated with excess body weight, especially the risk of obese children growing up to become obese adults with health complications such as cardiovascular disease, hypertension, and type 2 diabetes.[5] The vast majority of obese adolescents remain obese into their late 20s and early 30s. In fact, one study found that only about 10 percent of obese adolescents were not obese twelve years later.[6]

Warnings about childhood obesity emphasize the potential negative consequences for both the individual and society. In 2005, the National Institute on Aging predicted that the current generation of children may be the first who will not live longer than their parents' generation due to health complications related to obesity. In 2010, a group of retired military generals and admirals issued a report entitled "Too Fat to Fight," which claimed that about 25 percent of people between the ages of 17 and 24 are too overweight to join the armed forces.[7] Viewing this as a threat to national security, the former surgeon general Richard Carmona said, "obesity is a terror within. It is destroying our society from within and unless we do something about it, the magnitude of the dilemma will dwarf 9/11 or any other terrorist event."[8]

In response, a small group of scholars and activists contend that obesity is a moral panic that may be rooted in but extends beyond medical concerns. While acknowledging that the number of overweight people has increased over time, these critics argue that BMI is a flawed measure, and they contest the categories of normal, overweight, and obese.[9] The most notable example of the social construction of these categories occurred in June 1998 when the National Institutes of Health lowered the BMI cutoff point from 27 to 25, which caused millions of Americans to become classified as overweight overnight.[10] Additionally, they point out that the science behind the association between obesity and poor health is either inconclusive or incorrect.[11] Many question whether BMI categories accurately measure health risk, and there is some evidence that dieting can be more harmful to health than being overweight.[12] Whereas public health researchers argue that the solution lies in reducing BMI, fat acceptance scholars and activists warn that attempts to eliminate obesity may increase stigmatization of those with BMIs falling outside the "normal" range, and the solution instead lies in encouraging body acceptance.

In addition to calling into question the validity of the "obesity epidemic," recent scholarship illustrates how antifat ideology denies rights and perpetuates inequality.[13] The failure to control weight is linked to a host of negative consequences, such as poor economic outcomes, lower worker productivity, rising health care costs, threatened national security, decreased longevity, personal unhappiness, and passing on obesity to future generations.[14] This is the type of rhetoric invoked by Michelle Obama's Let's Move! campaign. By contrast, bodily practices that represent self-control are associated with personal qualities that lead to success, both individually and collectively. At the societal level, if children ultimately fail to contribute to society due to excess body weight, they are deemed bad future citizens who imperil the nation. The ideals and anxieties associated with children are often tied to concerns about the future. The obsession with children's bodies, particularly their weight, is not merely an aesthetic preference or a means of ensuring health. Instead, children's bodies are symbolic sites of meaning construction and contestation related to political and moral issues.

While children are sometimes targeted for education about obesity in an attempt to instill a rational, responsible autonomy that allows them to make "good" choices, children are more often the targets of public policy that frames them as vulnerable and in need of protection for their own benefit and for the good of the broader community.[15] Thus childhood obesity is often blamed on parents, school, and society.[16] The central tension in attempting to solve the issue of childhood obesity is between the agency of children to make their own decisions regarding food and exercise and the idea that children are innocent victims who must be protected from an obesogenic society.[17]

Public Health scholar John Coveney outlines three child subject positions in the antiobesity movement: sick children, innocent children, and antisocial children.[18] First, sick children are regarded as developing greater real and potential cases of illness than in the past. Portraying children as sick puts the blame on society for not protecting them from social factors that induce a sedentary lifestyle and overeating. Second, innocent children are regarded as vulnerable to the free market and society's failure to protect their innocence. Children are young and vulnerable members of society so they must be protected against risks like an obesogenic environment. Finally, the antisocial frame views children as problematic in both the individual and the social sense. In relation to childhood obesity, children are the problem based on their eating, fitness, and body size and for the potential negative consequences that they will bring to bear on social institutions in the future.

While past scholarship provides critical insight into how obesity is framed as a social problem and the implications of childhood obesity for problematizing children, these analyses leave out the lived experience and the negotiated meanings that children generate in their everyday lives. Instead of deconstructing cultural discourses related to childhood obesity, I ask how those discourses are internalized by children. What is it like to be a child whose body is labeled as "too large" amid a broader cultural panic surrounding childhood obesity? How do children find out that their body is a problem? Who tells them and how do they respond?

Today, more children at younger ages than ever before must contend with powerful messages that their body weight is a problem and that they must do something to solve this problem. The children at the weight loss camp knew about Michelle Obama's Let's Move! program and the many news stories proclaiming a "childhood obesity epidemic." It was within this cultural context that they had to make sense of their own bodies and the weight loss messages that the camp sent them each day.

Given the scholarly divide between those who view childhood obesity as a legitimate social problem and those who do not, it is important for me to explain my use of language in reference to the children's body size. The choice of terminology is complicated. Fat acceptance activists seek to reclaim the word "fat" and deem "obesity" to be a medicalized and offensive term. However, this reclamation of the word "fat" has not become mainstream,[19] and many of the children in my study viewed and experienced the word "fat" as a derogatory slur. Whether one uses fat, obese, or another descriptor, like big or plus-sized, "in a society such as the United States, where rates of fat stigma and thin idealization are very high, all of these terms carry at least some negative connotations."[20] For this book, I will employ the terms "underweight," "normal weight," "overweight," or "obese," when BMI categories are referenced in academic studies, at camp, or in relation to the construction of childhood obesity as a social problem. In my analysis and discussion, I will use the word "fat" in line with fat studies scholarship, but I will not use it as a descriptor for my respondents out of respect for what the word meant to them.

Embodied Inequality and the Obesity Stigma

Stigma occurs when people possess a devalued social attribute that compromises their presentation of self.[21] Social interaction is used to classify information about people's conduct, categorize them, and rank them according to social position.[22] The body, particularly physical appearance, is always an important part of one's performance and serves as a "sign vehicle" that provides both intentional and unintentional information. The meaning and significance of bodies are generated by society, and these internalized meanings affect one's sense of self and worth. A person who is categorized as a failed member of society will internalize that label and have a spoiled identity.[23] Negative stereotypes associated with the stigma also increase the person's susceptibility to status loss, unfair treatment, prejudice, and discrimination.[24] While being "thin and healthy" is a high-status cultural signal,[25] obesity is stigmatized.[26] The obesity stigma refers to negative weight-related attitudes and beliefs that lead to stereotypes, bias, rejection, and prejudice toward people who are overweight or obese.

Embodied inequality is the cultural system in place that ranks bodies based on their appearance. Bodily appearance has implications for inequality in social interaction and social inequality more broadly. In contemporary U.S. culture, the dominant construction of the ideal body is a thin, athletic physique. For females, this ideal means having a firm body that is not too muscular, whereas the ideal male body is quite muscular.[27] Given the importance of physical appearance in contemporary culture, many social advantages related to work, education, marriage, and interactions are bestowed upon physically attractive people.[28]

While thinness and fatness are frequently associated with other social statuses, such as gender and socioeconomic status, body size can also be considered as an independent social status. The valuing of thin bodies and the devaluing of fat bodies reflect status beliefs, the shared cultural beliefs about the relative superiority or inferiority of different social categories.[29] Research has found, however, that the importance of thinness varies based on social status with white people, the highly educated, and those with high socio-economic status being more likely to value thinness and have negative attitudes toward obese people.[30]

Judgments based on appearance directly affect interaction and lead to embodied inequality. Negative stereotypes of obese adults include laziness, sloppiness, incompetence, and lack of self-discipline.[31] Obese people perceive discrimination on an everyday basis and are more apt to report interactional mistreatment than thinner people.[32] Negative stereotyping leads to weight-based discrimination and inequality in a number of areas. For example, obese people are more likely to face discrimination during job interviews, have lower earnings, and get fewer benefits and promotions, and they are more likely to be fired.[33] The "obesity wage penalty" persists even when other factors like job performance are considered, especially for women.[34]

Indeed, the effects of obesity are exacerbated for women compared to men.[35] Women report both formal and interactional discrimination more frequently than men.[36] Obese women are worse off than obese men in both educational attainment and marriage outcomes, and they earn less income over time.[37] They are disproportionately negatively impacted in their experiences with health care, mental health services, romantic relationships, and their portrayal in the media.[38] Women are also far more likely than men to be body conscious, to diet, and to avoid social situations due to weight concerns.[39]

While the research clearly shows a strong antifat bias that disadvantages obese people, it is also important to note that these studies look at patterns and not universal experiences. So while obese people are indeed more likely to experience negative treatment and encounter inequality, not all do. Additionally, the research on inequality outcomes shows some inconsistencies. For example, some studies show that obesity is associated with poor psychological health, whereas others do not find a relationship at all.[40] While the obesity stigma has real consequences for many people's lives, my position is that there is actually a great deal of variability regarding where people locate themselves in the system of embodied inequality and the extent to which weight adversely affects their lives.

One problem with previous research is that many quantitative studies combine the overweight and obese categories or put everyone with a BMI above 30 into one category of obesity. Many studies on obesity contrast obese to nonobese people rather than looking at more nuanced BMI categories.[41] It turns out that the consequences of the obesity stigma are either nonexistent or lessened for those whose BMI is under 35. For example, adults with a BMI above 35 reported more employment and interpersonal mistreatment, and they had lower levels of self-acceptance than people of normal weight if they perceived encountering weight-based discrimination. On the other hand, people in the Obese I category (BMI between 30 and 35) had the same levels of self-acceptance as people in the normal BMI category. The distinction between obesity categories is important to understand within-group variability for a stigmatized group.[42]

Another important finding is that the impact of obesity on self-concept is not based on body weight itself but whether or not the person experienced weight-related discrimination.[43] This reinforces the importance of social processes and interactions which enact embodied inequality rather than any disadvantage that is inherently linked to body size. The age at which people begin encountering weight-based discrimination is critical, and research on the impact of the obesity stigma on children shows a powerful effect of both antifat bias and peer discrimination. For example, being the target of the obesity stigma during childhood increases the risk of mental health problems later in life.[44]

Children and the Obesity Stigma

Children learn the system of embodied inequality at a young age. As early as 3 years old, children endorse the dominant thin body size ideal,[45] stigmatize fatness,[46] and hold negative attitudes toward overweight peers.[47] Preschool children are significantly more likely to attribute negative characteristics, such as being mean, stupid, ugly, and sloppy, to overweight figures, and children overwhelmingly preferred the thin figure drawing for a playmate compared with the overweight target.[48] These stigmatizing attitudes persist among elementary school children between the ages of 4 and 11 years who also attached multiple negative qualities to obese targets, including being ugly, selfish, lazy, stupid, and lying, getting teased, and having few friends.[49] Another study found that 7- to 12-year-olds described overweight line-drawing silhouettes as lazier, less popular, less happy, and less attractive.[50]

One classic study from 1961 on disability stigma instructed over 600 children aged 9 and 10 to rank six pictures of children in order based on the appeal of their friendship. The options included children with various disabilities, such as a child in a wheelchair, on crutches, with an amputated hand, or with a facial disfigurement; an overweight child; and an average weight child with no disabilities. The overweight child was ranked as least likable and came in last as a potential friend by both boys and girls. In a 2003 replication study with over 450 children, researchers found that the obese child was still ranked last and was ranked as even more unlikable than in the original study.

Among adolescent and college students, the antifat bias persists but appears to lessen as children grow up. Overweight teen girls said that their peers commonly stereotyped them as being lazy, being unclean, eating too much, being unable to perform certain physical activities (e.g., dancing), not having feelings, and unable to "get a boyfriend."[51] However, older adolescents and college students rated larger-sized figures as more acceptable compared with elementary school children.[52]

Given the research findings that antifat bias and attitudes are prevalent among children, it is no surprise that children are aware of and internalize this fat phobia. The fear of becoming fat starts early, with 40 percent of girls in elementary school reporting that they are dissatisfied with their body[53] and children as young as 5 saying they have a desire to be thinner and to diet.[54] People who are overweight are just as likely to hold antifat attitudes as thinner people,[55] and this holds true for overweight children who express negative stereotypes of obesity at the same rate as normal weight children.[56]

As would be expected from the negative attitudes children hold about obesity, children are more likely to exclude and tease overweight children.[57] Overweight adolescents are more likely to be socially isolated and less likely to be nominated by their peers as friends than normal-weight students.[58] As BMI increases, students receive fewer friendship nominations, and obese adolescents are less likely than normal and overweight peers to have their best friendship reciprocated.[59] Obese students are less likely to spend time with friends, and obese boys are more likely to feel like their friends did not care about them.[60]

Overweight and obese children are more likely to be verbally teased, physically assaulted, gossiped about, or ignored.[61] Just as it was for adults, body size is a significant factor in who gets targeted for such mistreatment. For example, 30 percent of girls and 24 percent of boys report weight-based teasing from peers, but these numbers increase to 63 percent of girls and 58 percent of boys among those middle and high school students whose BMI was in the 95th percentile or above.[62] Still, it is important to point out that even at the highest BMI levels, over one-third of the students do *not* report weight-based teasing. While body weight increases one's susceptibility to peer victimization, it does not guarantee it. Understanding why some children are targets of bullying while others are not is important because weight-based teasing (more than weight itself) among children and adolescents is linked to depression, lower self-esteem, lack of peer acceptance, lower participation in physical activity, and unhealthy weight control practices.[63] In chapter 3, I explain how children negotiate peer relationships, teasing, and stigma as well as the varied experiences that the children had with their friends, peers, and family members.

The negative treatment of obese children has important implications for embodied inequality and the perpetuation of inequality more generally. Quality of life is lower for obese children.[64] One study found that obese children have a quality of life comparable to that of nonobese children undergoing chemotherapy, including physical health, psychosocial health, emotional and social well-being, and school functioning.[65] Overweight children do less well academically.[66] Obese girls are less likely than their nonobese peers to enter college after high school, especially when they attended schools in which obesity was relatively uncommon.[67] Obese boys, on the other hand, do not differ from their peers in college enrollment regardless of the school context. Obese youth are less likely to be accepted to elite colleges and universities[68] and less likely to receive financial support from their families.[69] In adolescent girls, but not boys, obesity is associated with lower educational and career attainment and more depressive symptoms when they reach young adulthood.[70]

Young people who are obese internalize negative feedback, which can lead to more negative self-concepts.[71] Psychologists Rebecca Puhl and Janet Latner argue that the research literature has not explained "*how* weight stigma is internalized by children; the degree that stigmatizing messages from parents, peers, and the media increase likelihood of internalization; and whether (and to what degree) internalization increases vulnerability to adverse consequences such as low self-esteem, poorer emotional adjustment, and unhealthy eating behaviors and weight loss practices."[72] My study of the weight loss camp examines the interactional processes through which young people internalize and negotiate meanings related to body size through social comparisons and attribution processes.

Stigma Management: To Diet or Not to Diet?

Erving Goffman delineated between a discredited stigma, which cannot be concealed from others, and a discreditable stigma, which is not immediately observable.[73] Stigmatized people continually face problems in social interaction with "normals," whether it is managing tension if the stigma is discredited or attempting to pass or cover as normal and dealing with the risk of being discovered if the stigma is discreditable. Obesity falls under the discredited category as it cannot be concealed. Although it is discredited, it is also predominantly seen as an achieved stigma, which means that a stigma exit is possible.[74] Therefore, the main stigma management strategy is transformation through a body project of weight loss.[75] Given the stigma of obesity and the value of thinness, it is no surprise that many people engage in weight control tactics. The annual revenue of the weight loss industry, including diet books, diet drugs, and weight-loss surgeries is over $20 billion, and 108 million people in the United States are on a diet.[76]

Stigma management strategies other than weight loss are possible. For example, some overweight men cope by participating in Internet chat rooms.[77] Online communities allow the men to interact with supportive others who characterized their bodies as attractive and cuddly or used fatness to signify a "real" or "natural" body. Alternatively, some people may resist the stigma altogether by "coming out" as fat and joining the fat acceptance movement.[78]

Finding fat supportive communities and joining fat acceptance social movements have, so far, only been available to adults. In her book *What's Wrong with Fat?*, Abigail Saguy argued that the overwhelmingly negative framing of fat as a public health crisis, immorality, and a medical problem leads to greater stigma, discrimination, and harm to people's health than the condition itself.[79] Yet even Saguy stopped short of endorsing radical fat acceptance when it comes to children. While she decried the fat-shaming involved with childhood obesity prevention campaigns, she began and ended the book with the complexities involved in whether children should be encouraged to diet or not. On the very last page, Saguy reflected upon the issues raised by a reviewer of her book who happened to be the mother of an overweight daughter and was questioning how she should handle her daughter's weight. Despite this reviewer supporting the ideas that thinness and health are not necessarily linked and that fat can be beautiful, she also knew that the social consequences of fat stigma are real. Saguy wrote:

> But she also recognized that she and—more important—her daughter are living in a society that values thinness. What should she do, she wondered, with this knowledge? Should she try to help her daughter to lose weight, not for health reasons, but so that her life will be easier? If body size functions as a form of inequality, should she try to gain thin privilege for her daughter? Alternatively, should she contest this form of inequality? Would it even be possible to make her daughter thin? Would it be possible for her to let her daughter be at the weight she is and not be miserable herself?[80]

Saguy did not answer those questions, but she instead ended her book with the comment that, "These are difficult questions. But the best questions are difficult ones. And good questions are better than good answers."[81] In chapter 4 I address the very same "difficult questions" that Saguy raised and explain why families chose to enroll their children in a weight loss camp and the processes by which the children engaged in stigma management related to both their weight and their participation in the camp.

Dieting Organizations and Weight Loss Camps

Feminist scholars have long critiqued dieting as a form of bodily discipline in which women are oppressed and controlled.[82] Others argue that women use body work, including dieting, as an expression of agency and that women are active and critical interpreters of dieting culture.[83] Weight loss programs also provide valuable emotional support and social service[84] as well as organized frames for people to deal with weight-related shame, either through avowal or contestation.[85] Dieting and fitness programs encourage behavioral and attitudinal change in order to achieve weight loss.[86] In her study of a commercial weight loss group, Kandi Stinson described how the organization's focus on self-help and view of weight loss as work provided structure and purpose for its participants. Yet ultimately the program relied on a willpower perspective rather than examining the emotional or disordered roots of overeating, which contributed to a high failure rate. Although past research has shown that dieting has important implications for behavior, emotions, and identity for adults, there has been little research that looks at the way children negotiate the meanings and experiences of participating in a weight loss program.

Encouraging children to diet raises the concern that it may be disruptive to physiological development or that it may lead to negative psychological outcomes. In 2002, Weight Watchers prohibited children under the age of 10 to attend meetings, and those between ages 11 and 17 needed permission from their doctor. The officials at Weight Watchers said that adult dieting programs do not work for children.[87] While their effectiveness is debated, weight loss camps are one of the few child-centered dieting options available to parents and children.

Exercise retreats and fitness resorts for adults date back to the 1940s,[88] but the first summer camp for children's weight loss was founded in 1963 by Selma Ettenberg.[89] Although the camp closed down three years later, Ettenberg soon bought land in the Catskill Mountains and opened Camp Shane in 1968; it still operates today. Camp Shane's location near Manhattan led to frequent media attention, including a 2001 MTV documentary. The camp can hold 500 campers and often sells out. Other high-profile children's weight loss camps include Tony Sparber's New Image camps in the Poconos and Florida, which can host up to 1,000 campers, and the Wellspring chain, which operated as many as two schools and nine camps in America, England, and Australia between 2004 and 2013. On average, these weight loss camps cost about $1,000 per week.[90]

Children who participated in immersion weight loss treatment programs, such as attending a weight loss camp or residential treatment facility, lost more weight than those in an outpatient or educational program.[91] Participation in a residential weight loss program reduced body weight by an average of 12 pounds[92] and led to increased self-esteem.[93] However, these studies are unclear as to whether increased self-esteem is related to the weight loss or becoming more self-accepting due to social support.

Children's weight loss camps are sites where complex cultural messages regarding body size, social status, and stigma intersect. A weight loss camp is also a distinctive context in which to examine how children take part in efforts to change their bodies while temporarily living apart from their families. An ethnographic study can provide insight into how children learn and negotiate inequality based on differences in appearance and body size.

Organization of the Book

The title of the book *Weighty Problems* not only signifies that weight is constructed as a problem for children but also indicates the heavy burden that the problematization of body weight is for children. This book has two main themes. First, I examine how children make sense of their bodies amid the construction of childhood obesity as a broader social problem and how obesity is experienced differently for children versus adults. Second, I examine how children navigate embodied inequality through interactional processes.

Symbolic interactionists have long been interested in how inequality is produced and reproduced in social interaction. This book examines how children learn about the body size hierarchy and locate themselves within a system of embodied inequality. Little is known about how children's participation in structured dieting groups affects their developing self-concept. Further, most of the work on childhood obesity focuses on how children may be impacted by their weight without ever talking directly to children about their experiences. This book gives voice to the young people who must both make sense of the embodied experience of fatness and confront the consequences of fat-shaming, antiobesity cultural discourses. By focusing on children we can better understand how individuals are socialized to problematize and manage their bodies in response to an embodied status hierarchy.

I describe the interactional processes of embodied inequality, specifically how children come to recognize inequalities related to body size and how they respond to injustices in their lives. Each chapter examines a specific social psychological dimension of embodied inequality and self-problematization, including social comparisons, stigma management, resocialization, and attribution. By examining why the children decided to participate in a weight loss camp in addition to their experiences during camp, this book provides an up-close account of the everyday, lived experience of children who attempted to alter their bodies through weight loss.

I find that the camp socialized the children to believe that their body size could be changed through effort and self-control. The camp's other messages, however, were often contradictory. The camp staff told the children to eat less but did not want the children to view it as a diet or for the children to develop an eating disorder. Weight loss was a top priority for both campers and the staff. Yet when confronted with the challenges of weight loss, the camp leaders told the children to focus on fitness and changing their mindset and habits. While the staff made attempts to address bullying and body image in workshops, the camp's education sessions also clearly linked fatness to poor health and lower quality of life. The takeaway message was that all of the children's problems could be solved through weight loss.

Because all the children problematized their bodies and some experienced exclusion and bullying at school, they viewed the camp as a place where they could be accepted and have fun *despite* their weight. The problem with children viewing camp in this way is that the camp's messages were not about body acceptance even though the camp was careful to not engage in overt fat shaming. By coupling the social acceptance at camp with persistent lessons about changing their body size, habits, and personality, I argue that the camp was just as psychologically harmful as overt fat shaming would be. By making the pursuit of weight loss seem like a fun way of gaining social acceptance, the children learned that problematizing their body was a source of bonding, comradery, and motivation. The internalization of anti fat discourse that had occurred prior to camp was amplified through the children's experiences at camp where they were told that their weight loss was a result of their individual efforts rather than the social control of the camp. However, the weight loss at camp was only short-term and likely to be regained when the child returned home. After learning that being a good person and having high self-esteem was linked to pursuing and achieving weight loss, the camp set up the children to become cyclical dieters and to equate their inner worth with their outer appearance.

In chapter 2, I provide a history of Camp Odyssey, an overview of the camp's philosophy, and a description of the camp staff and campers. I also explain my positionality and methodology, and how I negotiated the accomplishment of empathy during my fieldwork and interviews. Chapter 3 draws on the theory of social comparisons to explain how the campers learned to problematize their bodies through interactions with their peers prior to attending camp. It also looks at how gender is an important dimension in the negotiation of embodied inequality. Chapter 4 examines how the children decided to attend a weight loss camp, how their families participated in this decision, and whether they told their peers about the camp. This chapter also describes how children negotiated the potential stigma of camp by constructing various definitions of the camp ranging from a "fat camp" to a "fitness camp."

The next three chapters focus on interactional processes at camp. In chapter 5, the children explain their views on what causes weight gain and their own personal stake in changing their bodies. While the children had multiple attributions for weight, the camp attempted to socialize them into adopting the camp's preferred attribution that body weight is a result of effort and to reject other possible explanations. Chapter 6 demonstrates how the camp attempted to resocialize the children by not merely providing information about weight loss but also trying to retrain the children's tastes, preferences, and habits in ways that would come to feel natural to them. Additionally, the camp instilled a dieting discourse that connected self-worth and bodily control. Chapter 7 looks at the positive impact that camp had on self-esteem and how it allowed some campers to develop a more positive "camp self." I also interrogate the dark side of camp, including the complicated messages regarding body image and healthism that could lead to disordered eating. The book concludes with a discussion of the way the campers negotiated embodied inequality while at camp and confronted persistent injustices based on body size stigma.

2

Studying Camp Odyssey

On the first day of camp, I arrived at 10:45 A.M. to a long line of cars and the bustling activity of parents unloading luggage. I saw many young people wearing Camp Jay T-shirts, but I could not locate anyone affiliated with Camp Odyssey. I went to the main office to ask where Fay and Steve, the married camp codirectors, were stationed, but no one knew. I had spoken to Fay on the phone a few months prior to explain my research project and to ask for permission to live at the camp and interview the campers. During our phone conversation, Fay was warm and animated, with a folksy manner of speaking and a strong midwestern accent. She struck me as earnest and well intentioned. I explained the purpose of my research as clearly as possible, but I got the impression that she was uncertain about what an ethnographic study would entail. Still, she told me that she "loves research," and that I would be welcome to study the camp. While grateful to be granted access to the camp after recently being turned down by another camp, I was surprised that she did not convey any hesitation. I worried that she might change her mind once I got there if she misunderstood what I would be doing. We followed up via email, and she shared with me the information that she sent to the campers. We also negotiated that I would be able to sleep in the staff cabin, and I would pay a small fee to the Camp Jay directors to cover my meals.

I finally encountered an Odyssey counselor at the office and met Fay for the first time. Although she was busy managing camper arrivals, Fay greeted me enthusiastically and directed me to a counselor who would help me take my suitcase to my cabin. The counselor and I rode on a golf cart to the cabins that were allocated for Camp Odyssey. I was impressed by the massive size of the campground and how many campers it could hold. Whereas Camp Jay was a large-scale production with the capacity to house hundreds of campers, Odyssey was a tiny subsection with only two dozen campers and five cabins. The Odyssey cabin cluster included a handful of cabins for another separately run program for developmentally disabled children. I would come to find that the Odyssey campers were not only spatially segregated from the Jay campers but they also maintained an entirely separate social sphere and schedule of activities. While the camp programs shared a physical space and facilities, there was virtually no overlap between the two groups of children. It was like being on a field trip where several different schools visit a museum at the same time, but the students stay with their own group. We often saw the Camp Jay campers because there were so many of them, but we virtually never interacted with them. Over time, they became little more than fixtures in the backdrop to me.

As the counselor drove me to my cabin, he was eager to tell me about the weight range of the campers this year. They were expecting a girl who was 4'8" and weighed 120 pounds and a 12-year-old who weighed 237 pounds. He informed me that they had to reinforce the bunks sometimes and assign campers to the top or bottom bunk based on size and weight. This year, they had four cabins that were allocated to the campers based on age and gender (i.e., older girls, younger girls, older boys, and younger boys). I found out that most of the counselors and campers were from the Midwest. There were eight counselors total, and five of them were returning. The lead counselors, Chris and Taylor, had been Odyssey counselors for the past several years. One of the new counselors, Andrea, was a former Odyssey camper, and the other two new counselors, Wei and Sam, were college students from the West Coast.

After dropping off my belongings in my cabin, I returned to the office where they had hung up Camp Odyssey long-sleeved shirts and hoodies for parents to buy. The shirts on display were all size extra large. Fay said that she would get a T-shirt for me and asked what size I wanted. I said medium. A counselor told me I should get a small. A dichotomy between the thin staff and the overweight campers was immediately apparent, and I was being categorized as the former.

As the campers arrived, their parents were directed to a room in the camp's main office where they had to fill out camp-related forms. I sat at a table and told each child's parent about my project and gave them the informed consent paper that had been approved by the Institutional Review Board (IRB) at my university. However, it seemed that the parents wanted to rush through everything, and they did not pay much attention to the details of my project. Later, the parents attended a meeting where I was able to address them as a group. I gave them a detailed overview of what I would be doing, and I told them that I would be available if they had questions at the end of the meeting. The crowd reaction was positive and supportive. One father came up to me to talk about his interest in obesity research, and another set of parents was excited to tell me that they had attended Indiana University where I was enrolled as a PhD student.

The meeting with parents was my first introduction to the camp's philosophy on weight loss. Fay and Steve told the parents that their children would eat between 1,800 and 1,900 calories per day, and they would eat the same things as Camp Jay campers, only with healthier substitutions. Fay said that "the heart of Camp Odyssey is to teach kids, and the camp is an ideal place for intervention in weight management because the kids can recalibrate their sense of hunger and fullness here. People eat because food is out or they see a billboard advertising food. We are bombarded by commercials for food. It is mindless. This is why everyone in America has to manage their weight." Here, Fay conveyed that the camp removed children from the outside world where food advertising and kitchen cupboards induced the children to eat mindlessly. Camp, on the other hand, would be immersive and fun, and it would allow the children to change their eating habits and "recalibrate" their bodies without the temptations of everyday life.

In terms of effectiveness, Fay assured the parents that two weeks would be long enough for the campers to recalibrate and become mindful of hunger, but they would still be vulnerable. She advised the parents not to tell their children to finish their food at home because "it is better for it to go in the garbage than in their bodies." She warned that the changes the children made at camp were not anchored, and they could easily slide back to old habits when they returned home to a messy room and the familiar kitchen. She advised parents to quite literally change the home environment by cleaning their children's bedroom and even rearranging the furniture. Fay expressed her desire to stay in touch with the campers and their families after camp, and assured them that "weight is an up and down journey, and we don't expect you to be perfect."

The directors also promoted the camp. They asked parents how they found out about the camp, and a few responded by saying school referrals or the Internet. She said, "Tell friends about it. Camp Odyssey needs our help. The economy is bad, and enrollment is too low. It may be difficult for parents to talk about weight loss camps, but take some brochures and spread the word. Give them to school counselors. We want to reach more kids." They also accepted both corporate and personal donations every spring to sponsor camp scholarships. In past years, they tried to submit claims to people's insurance, but it failed. They told parents to ask companies to add a clause for weight reduction programs in their insurance policies.

When I speak to people about my research at a weight loss camp, one question that comes up frequently is whether the camp directors were profiting from the camp and how that might influence the camp's messages. While many weight loss camps, especially the large chains, are quite expensive and likely produce enormous profit for the owners, my understanding was that Camp Odyssey was not all that lucrative for Fay and Steve. Not only was the tuition lower than at other camps, but they had designated Camp Odyssey as a nonprofit organization. They also significantly reduced the price for a number of the campers, and they even entirely funded a couple campers out of their own pocket. While they probably made a small salary that summer and perhaps much more in years past when enrollment was higher, Fay and Steve regarded the camp as a charitable endeavor.

After the meeting with parents, we went to a large field where we played icebreaker games. I started to get a sense of who the campers were. The boys were active and sweaty and immediately started joking and playfully insulting each other. The girls were much quieter and overall appeared to be less overweight than the boys. Michelle told me that this group was one of the smaller sized ones in the past several years. The campers stayed in gendered groups, both by preference, it seemed, and also because the camp encouraged it by dividing the campers into three groups (older girls, younger girls, and boys) for activities. Campers were also prohibited from entering the cabins of the opposite gender.

During the games, we did an activity where we held hands and tried to pass hula hoops to the next person without breaking the chain. At one point, both objects landed on Janet, the largest camper. It was impossible to get her through the hula hoops, so she broke the chain. While it could be confidence building for those who did fit through it, I wondered if they took Janet's body size into account when planning this particular game, especially since she had attended Camp Odyssey before. This was the first of several times that I noted the camp did not accommodate Janet's size in the most inclusive way.

At the luau dinner celebration, Steve grilled hamburgers and hot dogs. Almost everyone ate a hamburger. The returning campers and staff commented that it was unprecedented to have hamburgers instead of turkey burgers. They also had lettuce, tomato, onion, pickles, and potato salad. Sam, a counselor, stood by the potato salad to help campers get what the staff deemed an appropriate portion size. I felt self-conscious as I served myself, but he said, "Perfect portion" with a big smile. At that moment, I realized that I was not going to be merely observing the children's weight loss socialization, but that I would also be subject to scrutiny.

After dinner, the counselors sang a song, "If I weren't a Camp Odyssey counselor, I would be a . . ." and then said things like carpenter, plumber, statue, and so forth with a funny rhyme attached. Chris, the head counselor, said he would be a camper and his saying imitated the campers, "What time is it? What's next? When do we eat?" I found this humorous because I had several people ask me what time it was during that first day, and I personally was thinking about when we were going to eat.

By this time, I began to assess the campers' ages and personalities. There were a few campers at the extreme ends of the age distribution. The youngest, two 9-year-old girls, were noticeably less mature than the others, and the oldest, Brandi and Candace, were 17-year-old friends from Texas who came to camp together. The two friends played games in the field, but they hung back from the group at the luau. Brandi looked tearful at one point, and she did not eat dinner. They sulked for the rest of the evening and did not participate in the face painting, hula lessons, limbo, or relay races. Camp seemed geared toward children between the ages of 10 and 14, and the majority of the campers fell within that range.

After a sandcastle-building contest, they handed out a "snack," which was a scoop of vanilla ice cream with canned pineapple and coconut on top. Serving hamburgers and ice cream on the first night was a way to put the kids' minds at ease about food. Ray, a returning camper, said, "Did you ever think you'd be eating this [ice cream] here?" The camp's approach was to intensely regulate portions while still allowing them to eat typical foods. The portion sizes were an adjustment for me as well. On that first night, I was slightly hungry at bedtime and woke up really, really hungry the next morning.

The History of Camp Odyssey

Despite my initial fear that Fay would change her mind and rescind my access to the camp, I found that she was supportive of my presence there. On the second day, I met with Fay and Steve and explained that I was trying to blend in and let things unfold naturally. I told them that I would mostly observe but sometimes I would participate in the activities and would be willing to help out if they needed me. They told me that they would not need me to take on any type of responsibility since there were so few campers. Fay said that she wanted to take advantage of having me there since it was a rare opportunity to have an objective set of eyes. Her self-reported "love of research" turned out to be true as she and Steve would often name drop researchers and reference research studies in meetings with staff, the education sessions with the campers, and when talking to me.

A few days later, Fay invited me to get coffee with her away from camp. My initial impression of her on the phone was only reinforced and amplified through spending time with her at camp. She was truly the dynamic center of the camp program, the one who led most of the programming and shepherded the staff and campers through each day. Her husband, Steve, played a supportive role in the background, but she was clearly the main purveyor of the camp's philosophy and the director of day to day life.

Over coffee, Fay recounted the story of how they started Camp Odyssey. Their daughter, Nicole, was studying nutrition in college and had been a camp counselor at a national weight loss camp chain. Critical of her experience with that program, Nicole suggested that her parents start their own camp for overweight children. Fay was an occupational therapist who had worked with marginalized children, and Steve was an exercise physiologist. Although satisfied with their careers, they were in their early 50s and wanted to do something new. Eight years ago, they operated Camp Odyssey's first season.

Fay viewed the camp as a way to enact her own personal mission statement, which was "to help kids build bridges to a better position in life. That is me; that is my life." The camp was her own social justice undertaking in which she saw herself as helping children to learn what they missed during their earlier developmental socialization. Fay said that she was bothered that certain children "don't have a fair chance in life. Camp creates a level playing field. The kids get in touch with who they are, and they like it. They come to see themselves as unique and wonderful as they are. They are trapped by their bodies. It is an anchor. By the third day of camp, they shed their self-consciousness and get in touch with being kids again." Fay's worldview was that overweight children were disadvantaged, deprived of their childhood, and that their true selves were trapped in the fatness of their bodies. The children who attended her weight loss camp were able to escape the injustices of their lives and recover a positive identity. They could reconnect with their childhood because after only a few days at camp, she believed they could "get in touch with being kids again."

The Camp Odyssey Staff

In addition to the two camp codirectors, there were two staff members, eight counselors, and two junior counselors. One staff member was Fay and Steve's daughter, Nicole, who was the impetus for Camp Odyssey's founding. The other was Nicole's childhood friend, Michelle, who had been on staff since Camp Odyssey started. Both women were thin and blond. Like me, they were in their late 20s. I shared a cabin with them, although Nicole rarely slept at the camp. Nicole was a registered dietician, and Michelle was a perky elementary school teacher who wanted to get her master's degree in counseling. She mentioned that her experiences with former campers who cut themselves in the bathroom and dealing with other psychological issues that arose at camp over the years had prepared her to go into youth counseling.

The eight counselors were all college students between the ages of 20 and 23, and they were paid $1,000 for the four-week session. They each had an hour off per day. There were two counselors assigned to each cabin, so they alternated evening duty, with one counselor staying behind with the sleeping campers while the other was able to socialize at camp or go to a nearby bar for a drink.

One recurring topic of discussion among the staff was how nobody could follow the diet of the campers. The returning counselors reminisced about all of the junk food they ate when off duty. Taylor said that she gained 3 pounds one summer because they ate so much pizza at night. Michelle told me that she tried to eat like the campers one summer, but she felt too weak to keep it up. She said that Fay had also tried it once but could not stick with it either. The counselors frequently made disapproving remarks about how the campers liked to eat junk food and "pig out," yet they indulged in the same off-limits food in a manner that was both self-conscious and fetishized given the near constant focus on nutrition and eating habits at camp. One night after the campers were asleep, they made elaborate s'mores using Oreo cookies as the base and ate so many that they complained of a stomachache.

The greatest staff controversy of the summer centered on Andrea, the former camper turned counselor. She was the only counselor who was overweight, and she did a number of things that displeased the staff. First, she allowed the two sullen teenage campers, Brandi and Candace, to use her cell phone, which was a major violation of staff policy. She told them that she was going to leave her bag and walk away, implying that they could sneak into her bag to use her phone while she went to the bathroom. That way, if they got caught, she could avoid blame. Because they were able to communicate their unhappiness at camp, Brandi's mother contacted Fay, and they left camp after lunch on the third day. Andrea was put on probation due to this incident.

Second, the returning counselors complained about Andrea because they thought she had failed to truly exit her role as a former camper. They perceived her as flashing her privileges as a counselor, and they thought it was inappropriate that she knew personal details about a current camper, Dana, because they had been campers together in the past. The general consensus was that Odyssey should not hire former campers to be counselors because they wanted to show off their new power, and they wanted the campers to like them, which created problems as evidenced by the cell phone incident. I noticed that Andrea tended to have a negative attitude and was quick to reprimand the campers.

Further, the returning counselors accused her of being lazy and inadequately fulfilling her duties. Sydney, a returning counselor, complained that Andrea did not do the exercises with the campers in the morning and instead sat in two chairs with her legs propped up. At one of the counselor meetings, Taylor encouraged everyone to be more active when the kids were doing their movements to set a good example. This was aimed at Andrea, but she did not take the hint. Sam, one of the new counselors, commented that he did not think allowing someone of Andrea's weight to be a counselor served as a good role model for the campers. Andrea grew increasingly unpopular among the counselors. This was partially due to weight prejudice, overtly in the case of Sam, and more obliquely for the others, who saw her as "lazy" for not exercising, rather than being potentially incapable or in pain during movement. The perceived conflict arising from Andrea changing roles from camper to counselor was probably just as much a matter of the counselors resenting giving equal standing to someone they had previously known as a camper as it was Andrea overstepping her position.

Personally, I thought that having an overweight counselor and former camper could be positive for the campers because it showed that people of all body types were welcome to be involved at all levels of camp. However, at a staff meeting with the directors regarding following up with campers after the summer, Andrea commented that she wished there had been a phone number to call for support when she was a camper because she developed an eating disorder after camp. She also disclosed her plans to get gastric bypass surgery in the near future to a few people. For those reasons, I was somewhat concerned about her potential influence on the campers, but in the interest of maintaining neutral relationships with all involved, I did not voice my opinions to anyone at camp.

The final area of contention and Andrea's ultimate undoing had to do with the counselors' eating habits. The counselors were permitted to eat more food and different food than the campers. Fay explained to the campers that the counselors were athletic and in a maintenance phase with their weight so they could eat more. Camp Jay offered a plethora of baked goods and desserts at every meal. Sometimes, Sam, the most ardent health advocate, brought around a tray of desserts for the counselors. While I was also allowed to get more food, I felt too guilty to do so and followed what the campers ate at meals, opting instead to eat additional food in the privacy of my cabin. In addition to the desserts that the campers could not have, most of the male counselors and Andrea ate bread with peanut butter to supplement their breakfast each day. Since I was eating in solidarity with the campers at mealtimes, I can attest to the visceral impact that peanut butter has on a restricted eater. Peanut butter has a powerful smell, and its sweet, fattening content makes it extremely appealing when you are eating bland, high-fiber cereal, a slice of cantaloupe, and a hard-boiled egg. I admit that my most privately contentious moments at camp involved my inner resentment of the counselors' unabashed spreading of not one, but two peanut butter packets on their bread. It is fitting, then, that a peanut butter scandal would be the final straw in Andrea's tenure as an Odyssey counselor.

Dana and Sharon were returning campers given the designation of "junior counselors." At first, the junior counselors were permitted to get extra servings and different food because they were regarded as being in a maintenance phase like the counselors. After the first week, however, the junior counselors were deemed to be abusing their peanut butter privileges because they were gaining weight. Since they were technically paying to be campers, the directors changed the rule so that junior counselors were allowed to get extra servings of what the campers ate but they could not eat the off limits Camp Jay food like desserts or peanut butter. On the tenth day of camp, Andrea overheard Fay, Steve, and

Michelle discussing how the junior counselors were violating Odyssey policy by taking packets of peanut butter out of the cafeteria. Andrea told Dana and Sharon what she had heard, and word traveled back to the directors. Fay, Steve, Nicole, and Michelle deliberated over Andrea's behavior, and they decided to fire her the next day. After breakfast, they gave Andrea the news and told her to pack her things, and she took a bus home.

Later that morning, they told the staff that Andrea had done some things well and cared about the children, but she had failed at other important things, such as confidentiality and not sharing inappropriate information with campers. Wei and Sam were the most surprised, but the returning counselors seemed to know it was coming. The campers, especially Dana, were shocked. The biggest issue quickly became whether the girls' cabins would be combined because Sydney would not have anyone to cover for her now that Andrea was gone. The girls were very concerned about moving their belongings and how crowded one cabin would be.

Andrea's firing also impacted my role in the field. The female counselors wondered if I could move into the girls' cabin and take on more of a counselor role. Fortunately, Fay never asked me to do so, and the girls' cabins were ultimately combined. Still, the counselors seemed to shift their perception of me since I could now fill the missing female counselor spot in their clique. Later that day, Bethany put her arm around a camper and then extended her other arm to me and said, "Come here, Laura, you're part of the family now." The campers were keen to talk to me about Andrea's termination and combining cabins. Kyra overheard them and said, "Quit trying to pump her for information." After Andrea was fired, I was identified as an appealing potential source of gossip for the campers since they knew I was always around and traversed the different layers of camp organization. While I generally felt accepted during the first week of camp, I felt fully integrated into the group on the day that Andrea was fired.

Methodological Approach and the Accomplishment of Empathy

Teenagers commonly complain that the adults in their lives do not understand them. If their parents and teachers "just don't get it," how is it possible for a sociologist to truly know what it means for a child or adolescent to navigate complicated and sensitive issues? I was faced with this dilemma during my ethnographic fieldwork and while conducting interviews at the weight loss camp. To what extent can adult researchers be empathetic with their younger respondents given differences in age and body size?

Empathy is often defined in contrast to sympathy. Whereas sympathy involves "feeling sorry" for others, empathy requires taking the other's perspective akin to "crawling inside someone else's skin."[1] Theresa Wiseman defines empathy in four parts: (1) seeing the world as others see it, (2) being nonjudg-mental, (3) understanding another's feelings, and (4) communicating the understanding.[2] Qualitative researchers are typically guided toward empathy through methodological emphasis on reflexivity, sensitivity, nonjudgment, and attentive listening.[3] Each of these conventions may be rooted in an eth-nographer's personality, but they are also skills that must be put into practice through interaction with others when conducting research.

Although there is some disagreement as to whether empathy should be conceptualized as a personality trait or a state, I accept Wiseman's conclusion that "the literature points to empathy being both. People have a disposition to be empathic, but whether they are or not depends on situational factors."[4] Although some researchers may have a more empathetic disposition than others, the extent to which empathy is attained for *every* researcher depends on the interaction. Variation in the accomplishment of empathy has important implications for data collection and ethics.

On the surface, it seems as though empathy would always be a good thing for qualitative researchers to practice. However, not everybody agrees that empathy is possible or even desirable. For example, Cate Watson argues that researchers often assume that empathy is achieved when they are actually projecting their own understandings onto the respondent and thereby limiting the depth and validity of their research.[5] Likewise, Patti Lather raises concerns that claims of empathy can disguise power relations in which the researcher feels that he or she knows more about respondents than they know about themselves.[6] In sum, these critics warn that empathy is a slippery concept that can be used to validate the researcher's worldview. In addition to the danger of overstating or misreading the accomplishment of empathy, many ethnographers face challenges while attempting to be empathetic. Although it is often expected that empathy for young people will arise naturally, this may not always be the case. Some youth may display personalities or behaviors that are annoying or disturbing to the ethnographer. Alternatively, some topics require contact with people whose values are deeply objectionable, such as when Kathleen Blee studied female members of racist organizations.[7]

Ethnographers bring their own personality and perceptions to their inter-actions. As one qualitative methods textbook advises, "Your ethnographic agenda, however does not protect you from responding as a person. You are still you, with all your own sensitivities, insecurities, needs, and desires. And any personal interactions have the potential to become problematic."[8] For all these reasons, ethnographers must recognize the dynamic emotions experienced during fieldwork and interviews. Given the personal and variable nature of social interactions in fieldwork, the accomplishment of empathy must be contextualized by the relationships and situations in which the ethnographer collects data.

Ethnographers' personal characteristics undoubtedly influence the extent to which they are able to gain acceptance and build rapport in the field. From an interactionist perspective, researchers are evaluated by their presentation of self.[9] Demeanor, voice, gender, height, skin color, and age are just some of the factors that affect how participants view the researcher and determine whether the research will proceed or not.[10] Ethnographers reflect upon how relating to certain participants due to similar background characteristics can facilitate empathy while also recognizing that shared characteristics do not guarantee an understanding of the similar other's perspective. Julie Bettie carefully considered her positionality in relation to empathy during her fieldwork that examined Mexican-American and white high school girls in her book *Women without Class: Girls, Race, and Identity*: "Racial difference was far and away not the only axis of my identity that mattered. . . . I often felt like an outsider around experiences of sexuality, family abuse, and class. At other times, I felt like an insider on the basis of those same topics. The logic of an identity politics in which identity is conceptualized as static and clearly bounded doesn't easily acknowledge the continuum of experience, relative sameness and difference, and degrees of intersubjectivity that allow for emotional empathy and political alliance."[11]

Thus it is important for ethnographers to remember that their social identity is not interpreted by every member of the group in the same way and that feeling like an insider or outsider is often in flux. Age, personality, and position as a researcher can facilitate or hinder building empathetic relationships with youth not only during the initial entrée into the field but also through everyday interactions during fieldwork.

Gaining Acceptance despite Age Differences

The night before the first day of camp, I stayed at a nearby hotel. I worried about "entering the field" and whether I would be accepted. My mind wandered to the worst-case scenario in which I would get kicked out of camp for being too awkward. Even though I was 27 years old at the time, I was transported back to feeling like I did when I started middle school. I told myself that the campers likely shared my nerves and concerns about acceptance. Fortunately, my fears were unwarranted, and I instantly felt comfortable at camp after a warm welcome by the counselors and spending an enjoyable first day playing icebreaker games with the campers.

One challenge of studying youth is gaining acceptance despite the age difference between researchers and youth. Although all ethnographers must develop a strategy to gain acceptance in the field, those who study children and adolescents will initially be marked as an "outsider" due to age, thereby restricting full access to and acceptance in children's peer groups.[12] When studying children, there is the unavoidable challenge that, as an adult, you are noticeably older and larger than they are. In addition, children and adults occupy different social spaces, and those boundaries are often enforced. Adult ethnographers may find their access to certain groups of respondents is blocked due to young people's fear of losing their place in the social hierarchy by being associated with an adult. Ethnographers of any age who study youth can use strategies to minimize social distance and gain acceptance, such as taking on the "least adult" role.[13] Still, researchers are often placed in a perceived or real parental role, which affects the type of data collected.[14] Age and personality can shape not only access but the type of research questions that one can address. In certain cases, younger ethnographers, particularly graduate students, may have an advantage in studying adolescents over older scholars.

The campers were initially curious about my age and asked me how old I was during the first days of camp. They typically guessed that I was 18 to 22 years old (like the counselors). When I told them that I was 27 years old, a group of girls remarked that I looked young. Since Nicole and Michelle served as program assistants, having young adults around who were not counselors was not unusual. Camp programs naturally set up a relationship between campers (those under the age of 18) and counselors (those over the age of 18 and usually in their 20s). In addition to supervising campers, counselors are expected to relate to and build friendships with the campers due to their closeness in age. My research benefited from the fact that I was only slightly older than the counselors so I could establish a similar dynamic with the campers.

By contrast, the camp directors were a married couple in their late 50s who had an authoritative presence as formal teachers during nutrition lessons and served as disciplinarians. The campers behaved more formally with the directors and did not share their thoughts and feelings as openly with them. Whereas the counselors had warm, close relationships with the campers, the program directors were more distant. Like the counselors, I lived in the cabins with the campers, whereas the directors did not. If I had been middle-aged during my fieldwork, I imagine that the campers would have grouped me with the program directors. Although I still could have collected data on the interactions at camp, I do not think that the campers would have been as open and willing to share their experiences with me if I had been older.

Accomplishing Empathy during In-Depth Interviews

In addition to three-hour-long focus groups held during the first week that centered on family support dynamics, I conducted in-depth interviews in a private meeting room with the campers during their free time. The interviews were semistructured, which means that I had a common set of questions that I asked each respondent, but I also followed up on unanticipated topics that respondents brought up.[15] Interviews lasted between 25 and 90 minutes. I asked questions about what they liked and disliked about camp, their family and peer experiences prior to camp, their perspective on body size and body image, and their hopes for the future. After each interview, I wrote down ethnographic field notes on the respondent and the interview[16] and a narrative summary of the interview.[17] Interviews were audiorecorded and transcribed.

One of the most common questions about my research is how my body size was interpreted by the children. At the time of my fieldwork, I was at the upper end of the "normal" BMI range. By asking whether I am currently fat or thin and whether I was fat or thin as a child, many are interested in how my body size affected my ability to attain empathetic relationships with the campers. Was I able to take the perspective of an overweight child? Did I have the emotional capacity to truly understand what the campers were going through and analyze it? Did the campers trust me enough to tell me about their experiences? The answers to those questions vary by camper. Below, I explain the general factors that led to creating empathetic interactions, even when body size differences were present as well as limitations to empathy. I compare my relationships with two of the campers to explain variance in cumulative empathetic interaction and point to personality characteristics of the respondents as an important factor.

Studying an overnight camp provided several advantages to building an empathetic relationship with the participants. First, I entered the field at the same time that the group met all of its members, which made me just one of many new faces on the first day. Being there from the very beginning allowed me to watch relationships develop rather than trying to understand preexisting dynamics. Second, living at the camp meant that I spent up to 12 hours per day with the campers, which facilitated rapport. The sheer amount of time we spent together meant that I had many casual interactions with everyone.

By living at the camp, I also experienced the embodied sensations of changing my diet, exercise, sleep, and social habits. I was not merely observing other people lose weight; my own body changed as I lost 5 pounds during my time at the camp. As I ate all meals with the campers, they knew that I was subject to the same dietary restrictions. During interviews with the campers, I could contextualize their descriptions experientially. It is hard to imagine being able to "get under the skin" of another if I had lived elsewhere and maintained a separate lifestyle while only dropping in for a few hours each day for observation or if I had only conducted interviews without ethnographic observation.

Furthermore, the camp encouraged both adults and children to talk openly about body image, weight, dieting, bullying, and other sensitive topics. These conversations occurred in structured settings, such as the morning education sessions on nutrition, workshops on self-esteem and self-defense, and informally over meals, between activities, and during weigh-ins. By witnessing and participating in these conversations, I was able to establish rapport with the participants before the interviews. The reason that the campers were willing to share personal details about their lives—and even secrets—during interviews was due in part to how self-disclosure and talking about body size were the norm at camp.

Finally, the campers themselves had a wide range of body sizes. Although I had not attended a weight loss camp as a child, I struggled with body image throughout my youth. In these ways, I was similar to most of the counselors who were not overweight yet shared information with the campers about their own body histories. My body size and body history, like my age, grouped me with the staff in the campers' eyes. Clearly, I was not a camper, yet I was part of a trusted inner circle. The amount of time we spent together and the normalization of body talk led to one camper remarking that "you get used to seeing people, and you don't even notice people's weight anymore." Still, it is likely that some campers saw me as an outsider due to my body weight. Although they rarely made comments about my body, one camper said that she wanted to wear a buttoned down shirt like mine when she lost weight. By making this comparison, the camper viewed my ability to wear a certain style of clothing as aspirational and indicative of my "thin privilege."

Despite the differences in my body size and age, I was able to collect rich, detailed interview data from the respondents. The amount of rapport that I had established with each camper varied based on a number of factors, including but not limited to my body size. I argue that empathy is a *cumulative* interactional accomplishment. Previous interactions in which empathy is established make it likely for the next interaction to be primed for positive connection and understanding. Likewise, negative interactions may cause people to go into the next ones guarded or confused. Conducting the in-depth interviews caused me to reflect on the quality of my relationship with each of the participants. I had gotten to know people's personalities and observed how they acted in a variety of situations. I took personality traits into account when gauging the success of the interview. Following each interview, I wrote field notes about the interview and the participant. Below, I share excerpts from these notes to illustrate how body size and personality affected two relationships prior to and during the interview.

Janet and Sarah represented extreme ends of the range of people who attended the camp. In chapter 4, I will use their stories to illustrate the wide variety of body sizes and experiences that are encompassed in labeling children overweight. At over 400 pounds, Janet's weight created serious problems for her health, mobility, and social life. On the contrary, Sarah did not face those same challenges:

Sarah was my first interview. She is 16, and she is also one of the thinner girls at camp. I wanted to interview Sarah first because she is mature and quiet. I feel like I can relate to her. I figured it would be an easier interview because she is probably motivated more by appearance than complicated health concerns or social trauma. This was confirmed in the interview. It was her idea to attend camp, and she wants to lose weight to feel better about herself. . . . The interview was insightful, and I got a lot of interesting information about how she constructed her body image through interactions with her family and peers. (Interview notes, June 27, 2011)

My interview notes reveal that I was comfortable around Sarah because of our shared personality traits and the fact that her desire to lose weight was connected to her self-image. In fact, I was so confident in my ability to be empathetic that I chose her to be my first interview. Due to our previous interactions at camp, I was reasonably certain that she would respond to my questions in a way that would allow me to be able to see the world from her perspective, be nonjudgmental, understand her feelings, and communicate my understanding of her position. I noted that I did not expect that she would share traumatic experiences related to her body size or health. Here, I was implicitly comparing Sarah with Janet, who I knew had a more emotionally difficult body history narrative. As expected, my interview with Sarah was straightforward, and I successfully accomplished an empathetic interaction. My relationship and interview with Janet required a different set of considerations:

Janet is 14 years old and 421 pounds. It is difficult for her to move around, and she can only participate in activities in a very limited way. . . . I truly cannot imagine the challenges that she faces or how hard it must be for her. The interview with Janet was probably the one that I was most apprehensive about when scheduling interviews. She is not very talkative and tends to be a bit sarcastic and cynical. I initially thought that she didn't really like me all that much. Over time, though, she has warmed to me, and we've had more sustained casual conversations about dogs and camp. (Interview notes, July 5, 2011)

Prior to my interview with Janet, I anticipated that I would have to navigate more difficult emotional terrain than I would with any other camper. Because of this, I knew that building rapport would be critical to executing a thorough, yet respectful interview. I feared inadvertently saying something insensitive that would cause her to shut down. Given our different life experiences and body sizes, I found it difficult to take her perspective, saying, "I truly cannot imagine the challenges she faces." Compared with some of the other campers who were talkative and effusive toward me, Janet also had a more reserved personality, which made me question how much she liked me in some of our early interactions. Despite my prior uncertainty, the interview exceeded my expectations:

> Janet is the perfect example of how an ethnographic presence can pay off when it comes to interviews. . . . She was very engaged and interested in the issues raised during the interview, although she did lose her train of thought several times. In fact, I would say that our conversation was the most animated and energetic that I've seen her during the entire time at camp. . . . She changed topics when I asked her about getting a new perspective when she gets older and lives on her own. I think this touched a nerve because she feels it is hopeless. She does not have money to go to college and does not have career aspirations. She doesn't have close friends and keeps to herself. It's hard not to feel bad for her and wonder if her situation truly is hopeless. (Interview notes, July 5, 2011)

I was pleased to find that Janet was engaged and open to answering my questions. She was particularly interested in a question I asked about how boys and girls are treated differently based on weight. I did not get the impression that she felt defensive or that any of my questions were inappropriate. She was a willing and interested participant who seemed to genuinely enjoy the interview overall. However, there was one exchange in the interview where I was unable to be empathetic. When talking about the future, Janet was pessimistic about going to college and pursuing a career. I was unable to take her perspective or understand her emotions at the time. I asked a follow-up question about whether she thought her views would change as she got older, and she changed the topic after replying, "I don't know." As I reflected on the interview and wrote my notes later, I considered "if her situation truly is hopeless." I could not answer that question, nor do I believe that I fully understood her life experience by spending a few weeks with her at camp and conducting one interview. In that exchange, I was unable to take her perspective and grasp the despair that she felt due to her family problems, her constrained finances, and her weight. Although I accepted her answer and did not press her on the issue further, I reacted with sympathy rather than empathy. As I listen to the tape recording now, my voice sounds compassionate and accepting, but my private notes are more judgmental and reveal my own perception of the distance between us in that I found it "hard to imagine" and "hard not to feel bad" for her. In these cases, ethnographers must strive for sensitivity during the interview, reflect upon exchanges that did not work, and be aware that variance in sympathy or empathy even within the same interview is normal.

Empathy is an interactional accomplishment that is influenced by personality, age, and other characteristics of the researcher. Even ethnographers with highly empathetic dispositions will encounter situations in which they are unable to take the perspective of the other, maintain nonjudgment, connect emotionally, and express this connection to the person. Given the interactional nature of empathy, it is important for qualitative researchers to take into account the variance in rapport, trust, and personality that occurs during fieldwork. Ethnographers must be reflexive and position themselves not only by social identity but with sensitivity to the range and continuum of empathy that occurs with participants.

Meet the Campers

On the first day of camp, I was introduced to the children as a researcher. During the morning of the second day, I was able to talk to them in more detail about my project. Nobody expressed concern or chose not to participate. Only four campers directly asked me about the project during camp, although I spoke to each of them about the goals of my research and explained informed consent again prior to their individual interviews. Most of the campers seemed nonchalant about why I was at camp. On the seldom occasions when a camper brought up my research, I sometimes felt caught off guard. For example, as we were walking back to the cabins from Bingo, I gave a drawn-out description in response to Zach asking me about my project. When I stopped talking, I could tell that he did not care very much and was just making small talk.

Kyra was the camper who was the most suspicious of my research. While walking to the dance, Kyra asked, "So Laura, you come to the pool with us and the dance and stuff, so what do you write about us? Do you write down what we say and our behavior?" I had informed the campers that I was taking notes, and my notebooks were visible during the morning sessions. I told her that I mostly took notes during the education lessons and that I came to the activities to get a sense of what the experience of camp was like. I told her that I didn't write down everything they said, but I was interested in what they said about camp and weight loss. When we got to the dance, I told her that if she did not want to be part of the research, the choice was completely hers and no one would be upset with her. She said, "No, it's fine. It's just that you have one of those faces that people trust, and people tell you all this stuff, and you could be writing it all down." A couple days later, a few of the girls were talking about boys and making sexual jokes at a picnic table. Kyra looked over at me and jokingly remarked that I should write down these juicy things they were saying. I smiled and said certain things could be off the record.

Overall, I felt like the campers easily accepted my presence. The younger girls were the ones who most frequently initiated conversations and physical contact, such as linking arms with me. The boys were not as likely to engage in conversations with adults, but they asked me to play Frisbee or basketball at the pool if they needed an extra person ("Ask the scientist to play," one boy called out, referencing my position as a researcher).

A few campers were particularly apt to seek me out for friendship. Three of the younger girls (Hanna, Faith, and Sasha) and the two boys who had social difficulties (Dustin and Ryan) spent the most time with me and asked me to sit with them on the bus or to ride roller coasters with them at the water park. As the most socially independent person—neither camper nor counselor—I was a particularly attractive partner for people who had not bonded with the others.

In the brief profiles below, I provide an overview of each campers' background, personality, and weight. I also highlight my overall assessment of my relationship with each of the participants. I divide the profiles into the three groups based on how they were separated at camp.

Older Girls

Kelly

A white, 16-year-old girl with freckles, glasses, and long dark hair with blond highlights, Kelly came from a middle-class family and lived in a small midwestern city. Her parents were divorced and remarried but lived close to each other and maintained a cordial relationship. Kelly was fairly quiet, but she became more outgoing at camp. She flirted with the boys, especially Tom, and seemed to enjoy herself during the social activities. Kelly and I often made small talk during hikes or while walking to activities. In our conversations, she made self-conscious observations like "no wonder I'm overweight" in reference to a knapsack with a cartoon Pop-Tart that she had earned from sending in labels from Pop-Tart boxes. She requested to schedule her interview during the last days of camp because she wanted to reflect on the experience as a whole. Kelly entered camp with a BMI in the overweight category. Her weight was evenly distributed across her small frame. Kelly stayed at camp for four weeks and lost 10 pounds.

Sarah

As described above, Sarah was a white, 16-year-old girl from a middle-class family. She attended camp with her younger brother, Jacob. Sarah recalled thinking about her weight as far back as 9 years old, although her mother only began considering it an issue over the past year. Sarah entered camp with a BMI in the overweight category, and she lost 4 pounds during her two-week stay at camp.

Dana

Dana was a white, 16-year-old junior counselor who had attended Camp Odyssey for five out of the past six years. When she was 12 years old, she was 30 pounds heavier and had been as much as 50 pounds heavier in the past. During this camp session, she was only slightly overweight with a muscular body. Dana was the most athletic camper and always won the competitions. As a junior counselor, Dana frequently felt frustrated and impatient with the other campers. She commented several times that her enthusiasm for camp was a facade and went against her natural inclinations and personality. Dana described herself as a Republican patriot who connected better with people over the age of 50 but "those people are dying off." Dana wanted to lose more weight and become more physically fit so that she would be eligible to join the naval ROTC in college and ultimately become a U.S. Marine. During her four weeks at camp, Dana lost 11 pounds, and she remained in the overweight BMI category.

Sharon

Sharon was a white, 16-year-old junior counselor who had attended Camp Odyssey twice before. Originally from the upper Midwest, her family lived in Canada due to her father's job. She came from an upper middle-class family. When she arrived after the first week of camp, Janet and Kyra (both returning campers) talked about Sharon being named a junior counselor, and Janet said that it was because "she got fit." Unlike Dana, who was cynical about being a junior counselor, Sharon was enthusiastic and jumped right into the social life of camp. Because she was a late arrival, I did not have as much time to get to know her, so I was surprised when she jumped at the chance to schedule an interview. Her interview ended up being one of the most forthcoming and revealing that I conducted. Sharon was in the overweight BMI category and lost 3 pounds during her three-week stay at camp.

Janet

As described in the previous section, Janet was a white, 14-year-old girl and the heaviest camper at an estimated 421 pounds (her starting weight was based on a recent doctor's visit because she exceeded the weight capacity of the camp's scale). She attended camp with her brother, Ray, and they lived in a small midwestern town. Even though her cognition and speech were slightly impaired due to the medication she took for her serious mental health problems, Janet was smart and expressed interest in philosophical debates. However, she frequently criticized herself, saying things like, "What a dumb thing to say" or "That is stupid," even though I thought she had a lot of really interesting things to say. Her mother once weighed close to 1,000 pounds and was in danger of passing away as recently as the past year. Because her mother had been in a nursing home for the past four years, Janet was the primary caretaker of the house and in charge of grocery shopping and preparing food. Her father had major anxiety, and the family struggled financially. At camp, Janet could only participate in activities in a very limited way because it was difficult for her to move around. Her hygiene was also a concern because she avoided showering. She only had a few pieces of clothing that fit her, so the counselors washed her clothes for her every other day. Janet was in the obese BMI category, and she lost an estimated ten pounds during her month long stay at camp.

Younger Girls

Bridget

At 5'10", Bridget was an exceptionally tall 12-year-old girl. I was shocked to find out that she was only 12 because she looked much older. Up close, I thought she looked like a 16-year-old, but from more of a distance, she could even have passed for an adult. From a small city in the Midwest, she came from a white, middle-class family. She was very shy and soft-spoken. Whenever I tried to strike up a conversation with her, I found myself talking a lot to fill up the silence. If I tried really hard to engage her, she seemed genuinely interested. Other times, she looked unapproachable and responded with a flat affect. Bridget was in the obese BMI category. After two weeks at camp, Bridget lost 3 pounds.

Mandy

Mandy was a white, 12-year-old with strawberry blond hair. Although she was good friends with Jenny and Ada, Mandy would also walk with or partner with other girls because Jenny and Ada typically gave preference to each other. Mandy was fervently complimentary and tried hard to be liked. Her friendliness and praise extended to me as well. Through her repeated compliments of my "perfect, white teeth," she spearheaded what became a frequent conversation topic between me and the younger girls and *about* me when I was not around (according to the counselors). Although she had a boyfriend at home, she developed a crush on Jacob. She was very interested in gossip and frequently served as an intermediary by telling the boys who liked them or whom they should ask to the dance. Mandy said her weight has been steadily increasing. At camp, her BMI shifted from obese to overweight. She lost 17 pounds during four weeks at camp.

Faith

Faith was an endearing African American, 9-year-old girl and one of my favorite campers. Because she was so young, her immaturity sometimes annoyed the other girls in her cabin, and they were impatient with her. She was short, wore glasses, and felt self-conscious of her belly. She spoke in a slow, sweet voice and sometimes described things in uncommon ways (for example, instead of "gaining weight," she said that she wanted to "stop expanding"). Faith was adopted by white parents after being put in foster care when she was 3 days old. She had lots of brothers and sisters (she mentioned "twenty" one time), most of whom were also adopted. She was in contact with one biological brother who attended her Communion last year, but she rarely saw him. Faith had been concerned about her weight gain since November of last year. At Thanksgiving, she was around 90 pounds, and she weighed 125 pounds at the start of camp. She talked a lot about monitoring the size of her stomach for progress, and she told me that she thought her stomach had gone down an inch in one week. Faith lost 5 pounds over two weeks at camp.

Kyra

Kyra was an African American girl who turned 13 a few weeks after camp ended. She lived with her mother, grandmother, and brother. She also had a sister who attended boarding school, and her father lived nearby. Her family lived in a midwestern city and were upper middle class. She was very shy and seemed unapproachable at times. I noticed that her unanimated manner of speaking persisted even when she interacted with her very bubbly mother during Visitors Day. I came to realize that even though she looked unhappy, it was not actually the case. She sometimes smiled unexpectedly and had a great, friendly smile when she did. When Kyra came to camp last summer, she made friends and had a good time. I did not think this year had been as good for her, but she claimed to still like it. Kyra was in the obese BMI category. Last year, she lost more weight at home for a total of 16 pounds, but she gained it back over the year. During her month at camp this year, she lost 13 pounds.

Hanna

Hanna was a small, white girl who turned 9 years old at camp. She was extremely immature, and both the campers and staff found her annoying. Although bright and imaginative, she did not have the social or attention skills that would be expected of a child her age. She took about eight medications, including some for her behavior. She often fell asleep and lagged behind during activities. She brought a lot of toys and stuffed animals to camp and talked about animals constantly. During our hike at the lake, she spent most of the time making really high pitched, loud bird calls and naming the birds at the park. She also had a worm friend who she killed at a cook out. Her mother sent her to three camps during the summer. Fay asked me after the interview if Hanna even knew that this was a weight-loss camp. Hanna was the only camper who openly complained about the food, and she was clearly not interested in losing weight (nor did she need to). She had a normal BMI, and lost 4 pounds during her two-week stay at camp.

Jenny

Jenny was a white, 11-year-old girl with pretty green eyes and a doll-like face. She carried most of her weight in her midsection, and she probably would have been the stereotypical cheerleader type if not for her weight. She had modeled in the past and wanted to participate in beauty pageants. Her middle-class family lived in a small town in the upper Midwest. In addition to her sister, she also had two young brothers that her parents adopted from foster care. At camp, she was best friends with Ada and part of the younger girl clique with Mandy, Jasmine, and Bridget. She also interacted with the boys quite a bit, testing out her relationships with them and flirting. Outgoing and talkative, she was eager to be interviewed and told me early during camp that I could interview her anytime. Her weight loss goal was to fit into a medium or large. She was in the overweight BMI category and lost 14 pounds during her month at camp.

Ada

Ada was an attractive, African American, 11-year-old girl who lived in a large midwestern city with her mother, who had a prestigious career. Her parents were "happily divorced," and she was one of the wealthier campers. Ada and Jenny were good friends, and she was a central part of the younger girls' friendship group. She had been friendly to me throughout camp, and she sought me out to ride roller coasters with her when we went to the water park. One day during an education session, she gave me an index card that described her reasons for attending camp. On it, she wrote that she had been bullied and tried to commit suicide, which she later talked about during the interview. At the end of the interview, I asked what she would remember most about camp and she said, "You. You were always just here. It was nice to have you around, and everybody liked you." Just as ethnographers may find that they gravitate toward certain participants over others, some participants may like and trust you more than others. Ada and Sasha were the two campers who most consistently and openly expressed their positive feelings toward me and seemed to regard me as a friend. Ada entered camp with a BMI in the obese category. After losing 15 pounds in a month, her BMI category shifted to overweight.

Melissa

Melissa was the only camper who came for the second two-week session. She was a tall, white, 13-year-old from a small midwestern town. She fit in pretty well with the girls, but sometimes walked alone between activities because she was not as tightly tied to the other girls who had already established their friendships. When I gave her mother the consent form for my research study, she told me that Melissa was an excellent swimmer with potential to be on the Olympic team. She was athletic and active, but her coach wanted her to lose weight. Fay asked if she overate or ate the wrong foods. Her mom said both. Going into the interview, I did not know much about her compared to the others. However, she warmed up to me quickly in a short time and was very affectionate. While other girls teared up in the interviews, Melissa was the first one to cry and need a tissue when talking about how much she disliked her body. During her two weeks at camp, she lost 11 pounds and remained in the obese BMI category.

Jasmine

Jasmine was a 15-year-old, African American girl who lived with her aunt and other extended family members in a poor neighborhood in a large midwestern city. She never talked about her birth parents, and she spent a lot of time at home alone, bored and eating. Jasmine's birth name was Sheranda, but she went by Jasmine at camp and at school. Jasmine had diabetes that was not very well controlled. She had originally planned to go to a diabetes summer camp, but her social worker referred her to Camp Odyssey. Despite her different class and racial background, Jasmine fit in really well with the mostly white and middle-class campers. Jasmine was the life of the party, funny and outgoing. She told me that she would fit in at the other campers' schools, but they would not fit into hers because there was so much fighting. Her school life was difficult, and the harassment surprised me because she was so popular at camp. The other campers genuinely liked and accepted her. Zach told her that he will remember her for the rest of his life, and he'll tell his great grandkids about her. One of my favorite campers, she would often call out my name and link arms with me to walk to activities. Jasmine was in the obese BMI category. She lost 7 pounds during her four weeks at camp.

Sasha

Sasha was a short, 12-year-old girl with long, curly hair. Her parents were divorced but lived close to each other in a large midwestern city. From a working class background, she came to camp on a scholarship that her mother got for her. Other kids at school thought she was weird because of her artistic, unique personality. Sasha was the camper I knew best because she always walked with me and told me what was going on with her life at camp. She often repeated herself and used strong adjectives to describe her feelings. She was also extremely honest about her past experiences with bullying and how she felt about her body. She was difficult to schedule an interview with, though, because she loved pool time and arts and crafts. Sasha came to camp with a BMI in the obese category and went down to the overweight category after losing 12 pounds in a month.

The Boys

Zach

Zach was a white, 13-year-old boy with divorced, working-class parents who lived in a rural area in the Midwest. His mother was a bit overprotective during the first few days of camp and called Fay frequently to check on him. This subsided after she saw pictures posted of him on the camp's website and commented that he looked happy. During camp, he was sociable and liked to gossip about potential romantic pairings among campers. Zach was in the obese BMI category, and he lost 18 pounds during his month-long stay at camp.

Jacob

Jacob was a white, 11-year-old boy with round cheeks and blond hair. He came to camp with his sister, Sarah. Jacob was not overweight and looked to me like an average-sized boy who was on the verge of a growth spurt. Both he and his sister said that he was attending camp because he spent a lot of time with his overweight uncle, and his parents were concerned that he was picking up bad eating habits. His family wanted him to be more fit and healthy. Jacob was not very outgoing, but he was talkative one on one. He was markedly less loud and aggressive than the other boys. I often saw him walking alone when we went as a group somewhere. Despite not finding a close friend at camp, he usually ate with the other younger boys, Charlie and Ryan. When he spoke up during the nutrition lessons, he asked intelligent questions. He seemed to be socially successful at school and struck me as an overall well-adjusted, happy kid. Even though he did not set a weight loss goal and was in the normal BMI category, Jacob lost 7 pounds during his two weeks at camp.

Ryan

Ryan was a white, 11-year-old boy from a large midwestern city. He lived with his mother, father, and 13-year-old brother. His grandmother also took care of him and was instrumental in enrolling him in the camp. Ryan was very smart, but he lacked social skills, which annoyed many of the other boys. Some of the counselors speculated that he had Asperger syndrome because of his behavioral characteristics. Ryan was in the overweight BMI category and lost 15 pounds during his four weeks at camp.

Charlie

Charlie was an 11-year-old boy of Mexican descent. Extremely quiet, he spoke in a very slow manner that was sometimes hard to understand. He was also going through puberty, and his voice was changing. After Jacob left at the end of the two-week session, Charlie had only Ryan to spend time with in the younger boys' cabin. Charlie attended camp for two weeks last summer and liked it so much that he wanted to stay for a month this year. Charlie was in the obese BMI category and lost 19 pounds in a month at camp.

Ray

Ray was a white, 16-year-old boy and the heaviest male camper. Ray came to camp with his 14-year-old sister, Janet. The two siblings had opposite personalities. Whereas Janet was quiet and depressed, Ray was outgoing and talkative. Janet said that people judged him more on his personality—you either love him or hate him. Ray was a textbook people pleaser in that he tried to be exceedingly positive and told people what they wanted to hear. He also did not seem to have a very realistic sense of his body size. When I was handing out the parental consent forms for my research, his father told me that Ray "just doesn't get it. I tell him that he is in the 100th percentile [for weight]. If you lined up 100 guys his age he would be the biggest." Ray often referred to his muscles, sometimes in a joking way (when we were doing ab exercises, he said that he could feel his "inner six pack underneath all of this"), and sometimes in a more serious, yet inaccurate, way ("I'm 320 but half fat/half muscle"). His coping mechanism seemed to be denial, which made him unique because many other campers seemed hyperaware of their body size. At camp, he was in the obese category with a starting BMI of 45. Over the course of his month at camp, he lost 31 pounds.

Tom

At almost 6 feet tall and 290 pounds, Tom was a white 13-year-old who carried his weight like a football player (which he was). Tom lived with his parents and twin sisters in a working-class neighborhood of a large midwestern city. Tom was the most mature and socially adept male at camp. During the education sessions and the focus group, he was the most likely to make eye contact and nod. Whereas the other boys were quiet or had behavioral issues for which they were medicated, Tom seemed more like a typical teenage boy. He easily socialized with the girls, and they joked around and flirted. Even though he was only 13, he hung out with the 16-year-old girls, especially Kelly and Sharon. He looked closer to their age due to his size. There was some gossip about the flirtation between Tom and Kelly toward the end of camp, but it never blossomed into a full-fledged, public romance. Tom expressed interest in being interviewed and asked me about setting up a time, but I suspect that he actually wanted to get out of certain activities. Out of all the male campers, he complained the most about body soreness, and he hurt his neck and back while tubing. Tom was in the obese BMI category and lost 25 pounds during his month-long stay at the camp.

Gabe

Gabe was a 12-year-old boy who lived in a small midwestern town. He was a returning camper, and he seemed to have the camp lingo down. Fay was very impressed with his goal-setting chart. Last year, he told me that he maintained his weight loss from camp until Christmas and then gained it all back. He described himself as being the funny one at school, and he did not get bullied. He was also one of the more popular boys at camp among the younger girls. Both Jenny and Mandy liked to flirt with him. Gabe was in the obese BMI category, and he lost 15 pounds over the course of a month at camp.

Kevin

Kevin was a white, 12-year-old boy who lived in a small town in the Midwest with his parents and sister. He was a returning camper, but he felt very homesick this year. He said that he had more fun last year. He was also the instigator and victim of many of the boys' pranks. Kevin was in the overweight BMI category and lost 7 pounds in two weeks.

Dustin

Dustin was a white, 12-year-old boy and one of the least popular campers. He lived with his working-class family in a small town in the rural Midwest. At school, he said that he did not have many friends and sat alone at lunch. The other male campers did not like him due to hygiene issues and they viewed him as "mean." He was on really powerful psychiatric medicine, and he left camp a few days before the first two week session ended.

In the next two chapters, I delve into the body history narratives of the campers and how they ended up attending a weight loss camp. Chapter 3 focuses on the factors in the campers' lives prior to camp that led them to learn the system of embodied inequality, problematize their position in that system, and decide to lose weight. Chapter 4 then looks more directly at how the campers managed weight stigma and decided that a weight loss camp was an appealing solution to their self-problematization.

3

Learning Embodied Inequality through Social Comparisons

Sixteen-year-old Kelly worried about what other girls thought about her body even though she was not teased about her weight or directly confronted about it by others. Instead, she was perceptive and sensitive to the social hierarchy at school and felt that popular girls were judging her, even imagining what they thought when they were looking at her.

> Walking down the hallways, I just kind of noticed that I was one of the bigger girls in our school, and it kind of bugged me. . . . Of course, the prep, popular girls are all under 100 pounds and sticks and wear the expensive clothing. . . . It's just always bothered me that they kind of give you those looks like you're bigger, but we're not going to say it to you kind of thing . . . just the looks they give you or in the locker room for gym. It just seems like when you're walking in the hallway, you have girls staring at you and she's looking at your stomach and your thighs. I feel like she's thinking, oh my gosh, I don't want to look like her or it would suck to be her.

Kelly problematized herself and her body due to her own thoughts and perceptions without others' direct social feedback. Kelly's story illustrates Charles Horton Cooley's looking-glass theory of the self, which posits that people develop a self-concept by first imagining how others see them, then imagining a judgment that the other person makes on the basis of that impression, and finally experiencing a feeling, such as pride or shame, about that judgment.[1]

According to symbolic interactionists, the self develops through taking the perspective of others.[2] Theories of social comparison naturally arise within this paradigm as individuals come to evaluate themselves as they think others see them. Social comparison is a process in which a person observes others, makes a comparison within that social context, and then discerns how he or she stacks up, which usually leads to conformity.[3] Girls use social comparisons to figure out their peers' body standards, which they use to judge their own bodies.[4] Body weight and appearance are linked to adolescent social status and pressure to conform to appearance norms.[5]

Using a symbolic interactionist perspective of the body, it is clear that the way bodies are regarded is relational, interactive, and dependent upon the meanings and values that come from the comparisons that people make. Social interaction plays a fundamental role in appearance assessment and modification. People use social interactions to determine how their appearance is regarded and to make decisions to alter their appearance based on the feedback they receive from others. This meaning-making process as it pertains to the body is constantly occurring and negotiated through social interaction and directly influences how people feel about their bodies. A symbolic interactionist approach recognizes that the way people view their bodies is an active, interpretive process that is ongoing and dependent upon the way that people define and interpret situations and interactions.[6]

It is also through interactional socialization that people learn the advantages of thinness and the disadvantages of obesity through the way that they and others are treated. Embodied inequality refers to the cultural system in place that ranks bodies based on their appearance. The valuing of thin bodies and the devaluing of fat bodies reflect status beliefs, the shared cultural beliefs about the relative superiority or inferiority of different social categories.[7] This chapter examines how children learn about the body size hierarchy and locate themselves within a system of embodied inequality. Specifically, I detail how children learn to problematize their bodies through social comparisons and the adoption of status beliefs that mark thinness as high status and fatness as low status.

Popularity at School, Social Class, and Body Size

Teenagers encounter social hierarchies and pressure to conform to the appearance standards of their peers.[8] Adolescent girls typically have peer groups consisting of girls with similar body weights.[9] Beauty, athletic ability, and social class are consistently associated with high status, popular groups in schools.[10] Both male and female camp participants believed that thinness was a prerequisite for popularity at school and being fat damaged their social status.

When I asked Mandy how she thought her life would be different if she lost weight, she replied, "the girls who are popular, they look for [girls who are] skinny and beautiful. I always say if I lose weight, it's not going to change—well it's going to change what they think about me, but it's not going to change how I feel about them. They don't try to accept you if you're not perfect. So if I lose weight, I'm not going to go there, and just be like, "Oh look at me, I'm so perfect." Mandy identified body weight and physical appearance as the key criteria for popularity. She believed that if she lost weight, she would get a different social reaction from the popular girls who currently excluded her based on her weight. Mandy recognized the way that embodied inequality manifested in the social hierarchy at school. Having been rejected, she predicted that she would resist membership in their group even if she did eventually meet their appearance standards after losing weight.

Other girls found themselves disparaged and excluded from high-status peer groups when their body size was linked to low social class standing. Jenny said, "The summer between 2nd and 3rd grade, I switched schools from a school where people looked like me. I was really popular. Everyone knew me, I knew everybody. And then I went to the other school and everyone was so small. I just kind of felt like a sore thumb." Jenny believed her popularity at the first school was due to the fact that people looked like her. As the new kid at a school where the other students were smaller than her, she felt like people made assumptions about her social class. She said that her classmates were "really snobby," and she felt like they were thinking, "Oh this person is probably really poor." Even at a young age, Jenny recognized that small body size was linked to being upper class and "snobby" in certain social contexts. Just like Kelly imagined that other girls were silently judging her body in the opening of the chapter, Jenny used reflected appraisals to form a new sense of self as she changed schools. Without directly being told that her peers viewed her as poor, Jenny made the connection in her mind between body size and social class as she moved from a school where her body size was normal to a more affluent one where she was larger than the others.

Kelly had a similar experience when she started middle school in a wealthier school district. In elementary school, she felt like clothes and how much money your family had did not matter. In 6th grade, class-coded body comparisons started taking place. She said, "Immediately I saw the tiny girls and their clothing and I was kind of like, wow they're so tiny. I think ever since 6th grade I noticed that I was just bigger than all the girls at school. I just never liked it." She explained her views:

I know they do spend a ton of money on stuff because they all have expensive BMWs for cars and they tan every other day of the week. Why would you waste money on that? Why does being tan make you look more pretty? I know most of the girls' moms are very health nut. They run. One of the moms runs an exercise boot camp place. So maybe they just spend more on organic healthy foods. Their moms push a healthier image. A lot of them were dancers when they were little, too. So I guess the girls who dance always seem to be really tiny.

Kelly speculated that the wealthier girls at her school were thin because their mothers were health nuts who exercised and paid more money for healthy, organic foods. These wealthy mothers also enrolled their daughters in dance classes, which reinforced a thin body aesthetic. Kelly tied thin bodies to wealth and gave examples of how the upper class socialize their children to be thin. The image of being upper class then is to spend money on cars, like expensive BMWs, as well as to cultivate a tan, slim body as a status symbol. While Kelly criticized their frequent tanning, she did not explicitly resist their tactics to be thin.

Just as Jenny and Kelly saw the thin, wealthy girls at their schools as distinct "others" who excluded them because of their weight, Melissa told me that she suppressed her personality at school and was ignored due to her size. She said, "Usually, I just won't talk at school. I would be loud and happy and everything but everybody would ignore me because I'm bigger than them. Everybody was so small. Like they were just thin. Little sticks. And nobody else was fat besides Kathryn, and now she's really small. So I'm the only big person." Melissa felt betrayed by her friend Kathryn who used her weight loss to leverage a higher social standing at school. When I asked her what popularity was based on at her school, she responded:

> It's not personality. There's like a lot of mean people. And there's rich people. . . . I'm like an outsider, I guess. Because Kathryn was in the other class this year, 7th grade, so I never really got to speak to her and she's turning into a West Porter. West Porters have Vera Bradley bags, penny loafer shoes, popped collars, preppy. She's turning into a prep freak. She was not a prep freak before. I'm not a prep freak. They would just make fun of my shoes, and I'd be like, "Really?" Now she's [Kathryn's] turning to the dark side. I don't have any friends at school.

Melissa perceived the status hierarchy at her school to be based on a prep aesthetic, which she rejected by calling them "prep freaks." Her peers at school read her body size and style as lower status, marked her an "outsider," and made fun of her weight and her shoes. After her friend Kathryn lost weight, she went to the "dark side" and began dressing in the preppy style. Since Kathryn only changed her clothing style after she lost weight, this indicates that a thin body was the prerequisite for social mobility within the popularity system. Melissa viewed herself as entirely excluded at school after her only friend had left her behind.

These campers' experiences corroborate other research findings that obese teenagers have fewer friends than their thinner peers. While the idea that youth perpetuate embodied inequality through exclusionary status tactics in their peer groups is painful in itself, the link between body size and social class also speaks to a larger system of inequality. Obesity is more prevalent among lower-income and lower-educated people, and antifat attitudes are strongest among higher-income and more-educated people. Some argue that it is not merely the case that poverty causes obesity but that obesity can also cause poverty because antifat prejudice can limit people's economic and educational advancement.[11] Furthermore, as the campers' stories show, the feeling of exclusion is experienced not only as bodily stigma but also as a social class slight. These girls responded to the body size and social class system at their schools by shrinking their personalities and feeling inferior. The cumulative impact of the internalization of these microlevel interactions may be an important mechanism for explaining the long-term impact of obesity on earnings and education.

Appearance and Femininity

Embodied inequality is gendered. Thinness is tied to the accomplishment of femininity, and appearance pressure starts early as a part of girls' socialization experience. Body weight has important implications for female identity, and the successful accomplishment of gender is connected to meeting appearance expectations through bodily control.[12] As part of the "pleasing woman discourse," Lynn Phillips writes that girls are socialized to be pleasant, modest, attractive, and sacrificial, and that "women's bodies are not the sites of active desire, but rather objects to be admired and kept under control."[13] Sharlene Hesse-Biber echoes this position in *The Cult of Thinness* by describing how modern young women engage in body rituals to express their self-reliance and inner control.[14] She points out that the food, diet, fitness, and beauty industries along with the media are powerful social and economic forces that systematically pressure young women into believing that their self-worth is tied to self-control, self-improvement, and being thin. Conversely, "women who do not maintain rigid control over the boundaries of their bodies, allowing them to grow, to become large and 'unfeminine,' are treated with derision in our society, and that derision is tied inextricably to the personal freedom of women. Women who are fat are said to have 'let themselves go.'"[15]

The enhanced appearance scrutiny for girls and women was evident in the harsher standards for the body size that would categorize them as fat. A few male campers pointed out that boys can be much larger before being called fat than girls can. Ryan said, "If you're a girl and a little bit fat they're going to call her fat and think that she is fat. But for boys, they have to be fatter to be called fat." Zach said, "I guess for girls, it would look way worse because you don't see as many overweight girls as guys." Even at camp, Zach assessed that "most girls here are trying to maintain weight and not lose as much weight. There aren't many girls here who are really overweight as much as me or Ray or Tom." In fact, this observation was reinforced by the composition of those who attended camp. The boys at camp were generally much larger and had much higher BMIs than the girls who attended camp, with only a few exceptions.

Overweight females were associated with negative appearance judgments in ways that were not the case for overweight males. Dana said, "Even I notice more if a woman is overweight than if a man is because guys can be stronger when they're bigger. They can be more sturdy as opposed to women who just look sloppy sometimes. Women have to carry themselves very carefully to be overweight and still look good. And men don't really." Whereas a large body size for men could be read in a positive way as "strong" and "sturdy," large women were more conspicuous and could be perceived as looking "sloppy." The gendered belief that it is a woman's responsibility to cultivate a pleasing appearance is enforced for fat women who have to "carry themselves very carefully" in order to look good.

Given the pressure to manage their appearance, it is no surprise that clothing was a potent symbol of the link between femininity and body size for the female campers. Janet said, "Girls feel a lot more pressure to be pretty and not be overweight and fit into clothes." Many of the campers equated physical attractiveness with thinness and measured both by the ability to wear specific styles and sizes of clothes. Clothing is one aspect of impression management, and many campers experienced embodied inequality through their inability to purchase clothing that matched the impression that they wished to send. Sharon said, "I hate going to stores and trying things on and like, this doesn't look good on me because you can see my fat. It's really annoying, and I just want to look good." Sharon espoused the belief that seeing body fat means that someone does not look "good," and she pointed out the frustration she felt in response to that belief.

Bridget explained that the emotional experience tied to clothing was what separated fat and thin people because "it's different from how other people feel because we can't fit into the clothes that they can." Melissa felt that it was unfair that she could not buy the clothing that she liked. She told me, "I get so annoyed when I'm shopping with my mom. Like I can't find anything to fit me because everything is small, and I can't find my size. I just want to fit in the small clothes. There was this really cute purple top that I wanted. It wouldn't fit me, and I wanted it so bad." For these girls, being unable to buy and wear the "cute" clothes that they wanted was disappointing and reinforced that their bodies were different because they did not fit into the clothes that were targeted to people their age.

Shopping for clothes reinforced the high status associated with thinness based on the way clothes are sized and sold in exclusionary ways. For Jenny, the challenge of finding clothing in her size was the first time she problematized her weight. She said, "When I was 9-ish, I started getting concerned with my weight. There was this one store called Limited Too. They had clothes that fit me. That was my Justice or my Aéropostale and when that closed down, I had to go to bigger people's stores. It kind of puts that thought in the back of your mind, maybe it's not that store's fault for closing down." In Jenny's mind, the problem of not being able to buy clothes at stores aimed at young girls was the result of her own body's failure to conform to the clothing, rather than it being "the store's fault." For many young girls, the discovery that the vast majority of clothing is made for thin bodies was a powerfully personal and emotional experience of a cultural system that categorizes thin bodies as superior and fat bodies as inferior.

Clothes shopping came up repeatedly as an automatic social comparison to the thin people in their lives. Kelly said that comparing herself to a thin friend motivated her to attend camp. She recalled, "Shopping with her and she's a size 2, and I was not. So trying something on would look awesome on her. I'd search the back of the rack for my size, and it wouldn't look good. It was tight or there are just so many reasons. I was finally like, okay I'm done with this. I'm going to camp." Kelly also used clothing sizes to measure her weight loss goals. She said, "I was one size away from shopping in plus sizes. . . . I want to get out of double digits hopefully and not feel so bad when I'm shopping with a friend." Kelly wanted to change clothing sizes not only to mark her weight loss but also to feel more comfortable when she spent time with her thinner friends.

Jasmine recalled being so upset about comparing herself to a thin friend that she decided not to attend a homecoming dance.

> It was our homecoming dance, and they told us it had to be a type of ball thing where males have to wear tuxes, and we have to wear dresses. And my friend, she is skinny as a stick and then she was complaining about her body. I was like, what are you complaining for? You can actually fit in half the clothes and stuff. I should be the one who is complaining. I'm fatter than a lot of these clothes and you're skinnier than me and everybody likes you because of your weight. I get picked on for mine.

Jasmine told me that her friend did not have a clue how her words had affected her, but she ultimately decided not to go to the dance. In this way, her body size influenced the type of experiences she got to have in high school, and she chose not to partake in certain activities because of her weight and her inability to find appropriate formal wear.

While clothing may seem trivial on the surface, body size and clothing were additional sources of stress during a time when youth already have to deal with the problems of growing up. Dana said, "Like it [weight gain] just happens and then you're overwhelmed trying to get this to stop. So it's another burden on your life as if school and friends and family isn't difficult enough, now you have this fitness thing that's a huge problem." She poignantly talks about the issues that arise that people who are thinner have the privilege of never having to confront.

> My parents divorced. My parents got remarried. I've had a crappy life AND I'm overweight so that's something I have to think about all the time too and worry about. I can't, you know, it's like, Taylor can go out and buy clothes and look nice and be complimented. And when people who are overweight go out and buy clothes, it's difficult. It's hard and it's stressful and it's disappointing and you don't get attention from people. You don't get complimented. You don't, you're not [pause] noticed. I don't know. It's hard to say that part. But it's just like, you already have your life difficulties and then you also have all these problems that you get from being overweight too.

Dana described how her weight rendered her invisible. While thin people can get attention and be complimented for the way they look and the clothes they wear, overweight people are ignored. For Dana, the stress and negativity associated with her body size exacerbated a difficult home life and the normal pressures of being a teenager.

The dieting industry promises a solution to life's problems, starting with the body. One facet of dieting culture encourages people to set goals aimed at fitting into smaller sizes and buying new clothes.[16] People are told that it will make them feel happy to fit into their "skinny jeans" and to drop dress sizes so that they can buy new outfits to show off their new, improved bodies. During camp, there was a lot of discussion pertaining to fitting into smaller sizes. The girls shared clothes and some had packed smaller sizes in order to gauge their weight loss progress. As our time at camp progressed, one of the most striking markers of weight loss for me was noticing how certain campers tugged at and adjusted their looser clothing and pants that were falling down.

On Visitors Day, some parents took their children shopping for new clothes as a reward. Dieters are often told to reward themselves with new clothes instead of food. Sarah's mother promised her that she could go shopping if she reached her weight loss goals. She said, "My clothes aren't fitting right. And when I go to the mall, I want that stuff, but I can't have it. My mom's like if you do well after a period of time, we're going shopping. I'm like, yes! If you do well, if you get to your set weight you want to be, you're going to get it. That's good motivation." Just as ill-fitting clothing served as a symbol of the inferior body, the attainment of a thinner body was linked to being able to engage in clothes shopping from a higher-status position. Attending camp and the other sacrifices made to lose weight were seen as worthwhile because they would have material—and status—rewards if they were successful.

None of the boys brought up shopping as an emotionally fraught interaction they shared with their friends or family members like the girls did, and only two boys mentioned clothing at all during their interviews with me. Ray noted his weight gain using clothing sizes by saying that he was no longer fitting into his jeans and his 2Xs were starting to feel constricting so he had to wear 3X. Like the girls, Charlie said that he felt excluded from buying certain clothing he liked due to sizing. He said that if he lost weight, he would "actually wear more clothes that I'd like to wear. I wouldn't have to actually look for large sizes. Sometimes I'd see a really cool shirt and I'd really like it, but it's too small." While boys also faced challenges in finding clothes that fit them, clothing did not carry as much emotional importance as it did for the girls.

Appearance ("looking good") was an important status belief for female campers that led them to see obesity as low status and thinness as a desired status. The type and size of clothing available in children's clothing stores is a manifestation of systemic embodied inequality. At the interactional level, clothes shopping led to social comparisons with thin friends who could buy and wear the clothes sold in children's stores. These experiences directly led some female campers to self-problematize their bodies and to seek weight loss by attending a summer weight loss camp.

Athletic Ability and Masculinity

Many at camp perceived the boys as being motivated to lose weight in order to improve their athletic ability. Janet noted that males also feel appearance pressure, "I think guys definitely feel a lot of that, there's a lot of like, 'Whoa, look at his six-pack.' If you're not some buff, tan guy you're never going to have a girlfriend ever." Thus romantic desirability was linked to the muscular male body, and attaining a sculpted physique like six-pack abdominals garners attention and improves social status. Still, most of the campers reinforced traditional gendered notions of the body. Ray noted that males could have a large body size and still be deemed athletic. He said, "I think overweight girls have it worse because to be a fit girl you have to be thin, it almost seems like. To be a fit guy you don't have to be thin. It's different. Girls have it tough."

Mandy articulated the idea that boys are evaluated for what they can do, whereas girls are evaluated for how they look. Mandy said, "Girls are supposed to look perfect and have like a tiny body and they can wear bikinis and stuff. But guys, if they're overweight, whoop dee do, can they play football? All that really matters is if they can do stuff." Ada concurred, "If the girls don't look like they want them to, ooh, I don't want them. And if the guy is overweight, can he do stuff? Can he play sports? Is he good on my team?" While the girls were referring to their male peers at school in these comments, the male campers, for the most part, did not find that male privilege protected their social status. This was due to two factors. First, the boys were far more overweight than both the girls at camp and their male peers at school. Second, they were far more likely to have health and behavioral problems, which compounded the problematization of their bodies and created social difficulties.

Many of the campers, regardless of gender, said that they wanted to lose weight in order to get fit, feel healthier, and have more energy. However, the boys were more likely to talk about specific athletic feats they wished to accomplish, like running, pull ups, or joining athletic teams. Another key gender difference was that the large male body could potentially be linked to a socially valued status: the football player. Ray said, "I know big guys who are star football players. They're more muscle. They're still big guys. I could be just the same guy as them." By viewing football players as role models who are both large and athletically successful, overweight boys saw the potential for their bodies to have a place in the athletic realm. Ray explained, "Football is one of my favorite sports. What I would give to be out there in my high school uniform. Instead of marching for the band, I'd be wearing a number 70—something on my back with the lights on me, the crowd cheering. Even if I was a total benchwarmer, I'd feel so good to be on a football team. I always dreamed of it. I can't do it though." Even though Ray equated his body size with football players, he could not actually play due to health complications that made him ineligible for contact sports.

Dana said, "For a lot of them, I think it's keeping up. They want to be athletic. They want to be on the football team, baseball, basketball, and so they need to be in better shape. And you know you could be overweight and play football, but you still have to be able to run." This was certainly the case for Tom, the most athletic male camper, who wanted to lose weight from his stomach and thighs in order to improve his football performance. He explained the advantage and disadvantages of his size:

It helps with stuff I like to do. I'm big. I like to box. It comes with the whole body strength. Football. Weight lifting. It would be way different if I was like 5 foot, and I liked all this stuff. It's easier to be bigger and taller than skinny and short. . . . If we're playing certain sports like soccer, it gets tiring going back and forth. I'll run the whole way there, but I'll be out of breath when we get there. Contact sports are my favorite, full out contact sports. Soccer is also one of my favorites, but it's really the agility the part that is lacking in me the most.

The rest of the male campers pointed out a number of reasons for being excluded from the athletics. First, a few boys had little personal interest in physical activity and preferred to play video games, an outlet for competition that did not require an athletic body. Second, these boys typically lived in rural areas or lacked transportation to sports practices and games. Third, they perceived themselves to be at a disadvantage because they had not joined sports teams at earlier ages and believed that coaches preferred more experienced players. For example, Zach quit football because, "The coach. I thought it was pretty fun except for practice [which] was really hard and it's every day. And when you get to the games, you don't start because the coaches start their kids, and you don't get to play much. Too much work for nothing." Finally, the boys knew that they were objectively slower and less capable than others, which could lead to ridicule by other boys. Ryan explained, "Most of the time, [during] the activities, I'm always the last one to finish the races or I beat only a few people. I'm not really, even for a fat kid, I'm not that bad. [But] the older boys are complaining at me because they say I'm doing nothing because I'm not as active as they are. I don't do as much stuff as they do, so they call me lazy. Even though I try hard, it just takes time to be able to actually get to that level of activity instead of just sitting on the couch." In competitive athletics, the boys discovered that there was no room for them to build their endurance. Instead, their lack of athletic ability was interpreted as laziness even if the boy was genuinely giving his best effort. Ryan believed that he was not bad at sports "for a fat kid," but the other boys evaluated him based on their own abilities and not on his potential to improve.

Even the boys who had little interest in organized sports noted how gym class forced comparisons of athletic ability. Charlie said that he wanted to lose weight to run faster: "It's actually that presidential fitness awards thing because I always got participation. Some of my friends got national presidential awards." All the boys were forced to contend with expectations of physical ability and athleticism, even if they lacked interest, access, or ability.

Several of the female campers noted that if they lost weight they would be more likely to join a sports team. Kyra said that even though she was not good at sports, she would be more apt to try if she were thinner. Sarah said that she would either get cut from the team or they would not put her in to play if she were on a sports team. However, if she lost weight and got in shape, she said, "I can try new stuff that I'll be more successful at." She was planning to join intramural teams when she went to college. A few of the other girls cited sports, especially swimming and volleyball, as sources of positive body image. While these girls expressed an interest in and appreciation for sports, they did not connect athletics with how others viewed them or as a means of enhancing their social standing in the same way that they did when it came to clothing and appearance.

The exception was one female camper, Dana, whose approach to weight was far more consistent with the male model. She emphasized her desire to be able to do certain athletic things and described herself as large, muscular, strong, "angry, violent, and intimidating," none of which fit within the femininity standards established by other older girls. Dana was radically far from performing traditional femininity, and this seemed like an active rejection at times. She referenced female body builders as role models and aspired to have their "gross" and "creepy" six-packs. However, she also seemed envious of the counselors who conformed to the traditional standards of femininity and had what she perceived to be "perfect lives."

Embodied inequality was evident in the exclusion of most of the male campers in athletic performance and sports participation. The expectation was that boys will play sports and do so competently. Lacking interest and ability in extracurricular sports or during gym class led the boys to problematize their bodies and to feel inferior.

Peer Victimization

Exclusion and social isolation were not the only issues that the campers faced at school. Many overweight children also face peer victimization.[17] Faith compared herself to her classmates and wanted to lose weight because she was teased. She said, "My goal is that most people in my class are under 100 [pounds] so I want to be under 100 [pounds]. And some of the boys are not that friendly. They always call me fat and stuff like that. So I just want to get less weight so they won't call me fat [at school]." In addition to explicitly being called "fat," Faith also compared her body weight to the other third graders who were under 100 pounds. If she were able to get under the 100-pound mark at camp, she would then fit in with the normative body weight at school and would no longer be taunted for her size.

Campers had various strategies for dealing with weight-related teasing and insults. First, some children chose to ignore it. Bridget said that other people "think that I am like really insecure about myself and they bully me a lot. I don't like it. This one guy in my class, he always calls me tubby, and I don't like it. But it's fine. My friend thinks it's funny." She did not say anything in response and ignored his comments. Even though Bridget said that she does not like this boy's comments, she does not fight back because her friend finds the teasing to be humorous and does not offer support.

Second, children seek parental intervention to stop the teasing. Jenny was also the victim of gossip and rumors about her weight. In one instance, two of her friends were spending time together when one of them stuffed a pillow under her shirt and said, "Guess who I am?" The other friend did not answer, and then later told Jenny what she had said. Later, the same girl told other people that Jenny would be a perfect match to be an overweight teacher's daughter. She also recounted this instance of bullying: "We walked to her house and as soon as her brother and sister saw me they started laughing. The day after my friend told me that her little brother said 'Oh, she looks like she should be on [the television show] *16 and Pregnant*. It looks like she is going to wear a bacon dress to prom. But watch out, she might eat it.' The three of them have inside jokes about me." Jenny's weight was ridiculed as her body was likened to a pregnant woman, and she was shamed for overeating. Jenny's mother spoke to the girl's mother, which created tension and subsequently ended their friendship. For this reason, the children rarely asked for adult help in stopping peer victimization. By telling on others, it escalated the conflict and created further isolation and exclusion.

The most common reaction was anger. Sasha recalled losing her temper after a classmate sent her a text calling her obese. She said, "I got this text from this girl who I don't get along with at all. I have no idea how she got my number. She sent me a text that said that I'm obese. That just caught me off guard. I called her and I cursed at her. Because I was so angry. . . . I'm not a cursing type at all. I mean if you call me fat or something like that, you crossed a line. And you're going to wish you never said that."

Ray learned to control his anger when he was teased about his weight. Ray explained that some boys would "call me fat just to get me mad. I used to really react to it a lot, but now that I don't—I just don't anymore. They're just making themselves look dumb, the way I see it." There was a difference between that type of teasing, and his friends who "like to rib me a little bit but just bro-type stuff. They don't mean it in a mean way at all." Rather than getting angry, Jasmine used her classmates' taunts that she was fat to motivate her to lose weight. She said, "I think like this, for every one pound that I lose, that's one less person talking trash about me in my ear. So far, I lost 15 pounds, so I lost 15 people in my ear. By gaining one pound back, I gained one person in my ear."

In one case, weight-related torment led to serious emotional consequences for the victim. During many informal conversations at camp and our formal interview, Ada reported constant bullying at her school. The other students called her "fat" and "muffin top." A few girls posted a note on Facebook with Ada's initials that described her as fat and stupid. She printed the note and gave it to the principal, who suspended the girls who wrote it. Ada internalized the messages that her peers sent about her body and was brutally harsh in her self-assessment. When some of her friends defended her by saying she was not fat, she told them, "I know I am. I'm the average weight for a high schooler. A male high schooler. And they'd say 'Oh.' And I'd say, 'Yeah, that's what I thought. Don't try to sugarcoat it, and say you're not, you're not. It's like, 'Well guess what? I am, I am, I am. It's time to face the facts.' They said, 'Ada you're not this, you're not that.' I said, 'That's lies. I am.'"

Ada's self-concept was influenced by the comparison of her body weight at 12 years old to an older, male body. When her friends tried to counter the problematization of her body by telling her that she was not fat, Ada refused to believe them and said that they were lying. In her view, she deserved the "fat" label because her body was objectively larger than her peers' bodies and people confronted her about it. The bullying became so unbearable that Ada attempted suicide. She explained, "Around the beginning of 6th grade, I was really depressed because I felt like no one liked me because I kept being made fun of. I tried to drown myself in the bathtub. . . . My mom came in and saw me and pulled me out. She was crying and said, 'Why are you trying to do that?' I said, 'Nobody likes me and I keep getting called names. I hate myself. I just want to die.'"

The name calling and teasing were so damaging to Ada's self-image and emotional health that she no longer wanted to live. In addition to enrolling her in counseling, her mother decided to send her to the weight loss camp that summer and pay for private school in the fall. Ada was looking forward to starting over at a school where uniforms were required because she thought there might be less appearance pressure. Still, she hoped to lose weight over the summer. When I asked her how she thought her life might be different if she lost weight, she responded: "I wouldn't get stares. I get stared at a lot. I'm like why are you staring at me? Do I have something on my face, in my teeth? Also, toward dating, I might not be called ugly by any boys anymore. If they have something to say, they will keep it to themselves. They would always say it to my face, 'You're fat, you're ugly, you're stupid.' It's like well keep it to yourself. Maybe I am fat, oh well. You can't just like keep calling me [names] and think it's going away. It's not going to. So that." Ada was so convinced of the obviousness of her body size that she countered the bullies with the same avowal tactics that she used with her friends. She pointed out to those who tormented her that name calling was not going to change her body weight. However, she knew that the only way that they would cease bullying her was if she actually lost weight. In terms of embodied inequality, Ada articulated how she viewed thinness as privilege and a shield against taunts.

Social interactions with peers at school led many campers to problematize their bodies. They experienced firsthand the embodied inequality that stems from ranking bodies and the social rewards bestowed upon those who are thin. Some were targets of ridicule because of their body size, whereas others felt excluded, and they internalized their comparatively low social standing. However, as I pointed out in chapter 1, not all campers experienced bullying or peer victimization. In the next section, I explain how campers viewed and experienced bullying in gendered ways, and I discuss some of the protective factors against being the victim of weight-based bullying.

Gender and Bullying

While girls and women report experiencing body weight discrimination more frequently than boys and men do,[18] there were different perspectives among the campers as to whether boys or girls were more likely to get teased about their weight. Some held the position that people were less likely to make fun of girls because they were more sensitive and likely to be protected. Zach said, "I've only seen the boys' end of people making fun of people, so boys don't make fun of girls for being overweight." Bridget believed that girls may be protected from teasing because of their feminine status. She said, "I think people would be more mean to the guy because guys don't really care. If you're mean to a girl, it's not cool. They would just ignore the girl and tease the boy." Jenny believed boys had better strategies for dealing with teasing and that "girls when they're overweight, they're more sensitive about it. Guys kind of make fun of [themselves] or find someone who is bigger than them and make fun of them." However, Jasmine said that being overweight was harder for girls: "No matter what a boy do, they still get along with other boys. It's a thing about females. They think we are ugly and nasty looking and this and that. Whoa, I am right here. I can hear you. Nobody cares about what an overweight boy looks like. It's always about overweight girls that everybody has something to say about. I mean, everybody. I'm not the prettiest person in the group, but I'm still standing right here, you know, a human being that can hear every word you say." Jasmine's quote reflects what Jeanine Gailey calls the hyper (in)visibility of fat women.[19] Her body size's visibility marked her as a target for people to call her "ugly and nasty looking" while at the same time she was rendered invisible and dehumanized because they taunted her as if she was not there and as if their words did not affect her.

Faith believed that girls were subject to more verbal harassment, whereas boys were more likely to have physical altercations. She explained, "Probably a lot of the skinny girls or popular girls that everybody loves and their two sidekicks or whatever, if someone fat was walking the hall, they would just call out to everyone that she is so fat. They could humiliate her just because she is fat. I don't think boys would yell out in the hall telling everybody that a boy is overweight or like humiliate them. They would fight violently or something like that, but I don't think they would do anything the girls would do." Faith viewed girls as perpetrating emotional abuse, such as public humiliation and verbal taunts. Boys, on the other hand, would be less likely to call attention to an overweight boy, but they may be more susceptible to physical fights.

Charlie thought that being a larger size could be an advantage to prevent that type of physical bullying. He said, "The people who are teasing actually get scared because they get right up in their face" whereas girls were less likely to physically defend themselves. This was the case for Tom who used his size to defend himself against an older male who teased him about his weight.

TOM: I had a problem recently when someone came up to me that didn't even know me and said something. I wound up getting in a fight with the kid because it really set me off. I have no problem with my friends making fat jokes because I've known them for years, and we can make jokes about each other. But when someone comes up to you who doesn't even know you, doesn't even know your name, and they have no idea what you've been through, they really need to look at themselves. Like why would you say something like that if you don't even know the person?

LB: So you hit him?

TOM: Yeah, I got really aggravated and said, "You don't even know me. Why are you saying that?" And he got really cocky and pushed me back, and it escalated from that. The kid was 17, and I have no problem fighting a 17-year-old. Guys have gotten in my face before. Just because you're 17 and older than me, I'll still win. Because I am bigger. I am way more in shape than you. I can do a lot more than you. I'm faster than you.

For Tom, his size made him both vulnerable to being targeted by fat jokes and intimidating because he would use his size to physically dominate boys who were older than him. Despite only being 13 years old, Tom fought people who were 17 years old. Tom repeatedly drew a line between people who knew him and those who did not. If a stranger made a comment about his body size, Tom reacted angrily and fought the person. On the other hand, if a friend made a fat joke, he let it slide because they had established a relationship in which they engaged in mutual banter and put-downs. Research on bullying in schools shows that students take into account the intentions of the perpetrator and whether they consider that person a friend when defining whether a potentially negative peer interaction counts as bullying.[20]

Boys who did not perform gender in ways that were accepted by their peers risked being teased for both their body weight and their sexual orientation. Ryan said his weight affected how other people saw him. He said, "An easy one is when they call me fat. If I'm not fat, why would they call me fat? It would just look ridiculous to call me fat when I'm skinny." While it was seemingly self-evident to Ryan that only fat people are made fun of for being fat, he could not understand why he was being called gay when he was not. This bothered him more than the weight-related teasing. "It's just so many people are calling me that and acting like it. It's just not who I am. People can call me fat, I don't mind. I am fat. If I lose weight and they call me fat, I can say I'm skinnier than they are. They can call me dumb. I'm one of the smartest kids in my class. They are even dumber than I am. But when they call me gay, it's not true. It makes me so angry because of all the times that people are saying or act like I'm gay." Ryan viewed teasing related to being fat or dumb as something he could change or discredit. He could prove to others that he was smart or he could lose weight in order to no longer be called fat. However, he felt like being called gay was unfair because it was not his identity. However, it may be the case that Ryan was taking the accusations of being gay literally when that was not necessarily what the bullies meant. Sociologist C. J. Pascoe found that adolescent males often use slurs like "fag" to regulate gender boundaries and enforce hegemonic masculinity rather than to tease someone who they know identifies as gay. Overweight males, like Ryan, may be vulnerable to their masculinity being impugned if they are unable to compensate or prove their masculinity in other arenas, such as being aggressive or athletic like Tom. Likewise, Sarah talked about how the successful performance of masculinity allowed males to escape body scrutiny from most of their male peers. She said, "Most guys just don't tend to care. They're like, well, *you act like a guy*, you look like one, you're fine." Whereas even a small amount of fatness could spoil a girl's femininity, competently performing masculinity shielded overweight boys from losing social status.

Overweight and obese adolescents are more likely than their thinner peers to be teased and bullied. However, not all overweight or obese youth experience peer victimization. Even among my small sample of weight loss campers, a group that was likely more stigmatized than noncampers, there was great variability in the incidence and extent of bullying. The two factors that had the greatest impact on whether or not a child was bullied were how heavy the child was and whether there were emotional, mental, or behavioral issues present.

The campers who were not overtly or consistently bullied were Sarah, Jacob, Kelly, Kyra, Mandy, Charlie, Dana, Sharon, Gabe, Tom, and Janet. In general, members of this group were more likely to be in the normal or overweight BMI categories, have quiet personalities, attend small schools with less of a clique structure, and not have mental health issues. Janet was an outlier, but she explained that there was a "veil of respect" afforded to her by other students, likely because her large size evoked sympathy or pity from others. She also kept a low profile and was socially isolated. Janet said, "At school, I have no close friends. I'm not the kind of person who goes over to people's house or invites people to my house. I can go an entire day without talking. I come from a school—I am mercifully not one of the people that is ever picked on. Some people are and that is terrible, and I feel bad about it." Even though she was not bullied, she was not socially accepted. Tom and Sharon recalled instances of people making weight-based comments, but they both had large groups of friends, seemed relatively popular, and did not report intense or consistent taunts.

The campers who reported weight-based peer victimization typically had other issues that made them social outsiders. These coinciding factors made the child more of a target and exacerbated the weight-based mistreatment. Zach, Bridget, Ryan, Faith, Ray, Jenny, Ada, Melissa, Jasmine, Sasha, Gabe, Dustin, and Kevin reported being bullied. Members of this group were more likely to be in the obese BMI category, take medications for mental health issues, and have less appealing personalities. In a few cases, they were unable to follow the norms of social interaction or they mistreated other students. Although Ada was the recipient of brutal treatment by her peers, she also admitted that she was sometimes the instigator of teasing. She said, "I can be kind of mean back home. Sometimes I'm just like ugh leave me alone. And then I have picked on some people too. Putting my anger on them, and I end up saying I'm so sorry. I know how it feels."

Some of the campers noted that they were treated differently from other overweight children at their school. Ryan said, "There's a guy who is this size. He is short and he is fat and very funny. He doesn't get teased at all." Jasmine said that other overweight people at her school "get treated more fairly than I do for some reason." When I asked her why she thinks that is, she replied, "I don't know. I truly don't know." There is no doubt that these children's weight was a central reason why they were teased. However, the scorn they received for their weight and appearance was also a way of rejecting behavior and personalities that deviated from the norm. The harassment that many received was not solely based on their body size, although it was rooted in and manifested itself through antifat rhetoric and discrimination. Rather, it seems as though this group was rejected for both their fatness and their disliked interactional styles, even though the teasing was mostly weight based.

Having a high BMI raised the probability of being targeted, but it did not guarantee it. In contrast, Mandy and Charlie were both in the obese BMI category but did not experience weight-based teasing, which seemed to be due to their school's structure and their social proficiency. Mandy put forth a lot of interactional effort to be liked; she was always effusive and complimentary to others. Charlie attended a small school where he was quiet and unassuming. The variability of peer-based victimization reinforces the fact that embodied inequality is an interactional process. Having a larger body in a culture that values thinness makes one highly susceptible to antifat prejudice and discrimination. Yet the lived everyday experience and the level of trauma inflicted upon fat children often coincide with other compounding factors.

Dating and Romantic Relationships

Campers also acknowledged the dating difficulties faced by obese teens. Young adults judge both obese males and females as less attractive, less likely to be dating, and more deserving of an overweight, less attractive dating partner than thin adolescents.[21] Some studies show that obese adolescents are indeed less likely to date than their peers, and this dating penalty is more pronounced for girls.[22] Fifty percent of overweight girls in grades 9 through 12 reported never having dated compared to 20 percent of their thin classmates,[23] yet this was not the case for boys.[24] Many girls perceive that the importance of thinness to attractiveness affects their popularity and desirability to boys.[25]

For Sharon, feeling desired by males and being happy were related to being a lower weight. She compared herself to a time when she was both thinner and happier. She said, "I was at this certain weight, such a good weight, 130 pounds, a really good size. I had a boyfriend, and a bunch of other guys wanted me. I felt like I was happy at that point so it's kind of like, I compare myself to then all the time. I always think back to then. That's where I want to be. It's not really working." She believed that if she could return to that weight, she would easily have a boyfriend, and her confidence would also return.

Part of the pressure she felt to lose weight in order to have a boyfriend was related to a gendered double standard on the dating market. Sharon said, "I find that when it comes to getting guys, guys judge girls on your body usually, most guys, not all of them. Most guys in the world judge girls on their looks. But girls aren't always like that. They have more feelings and they judge on personality." Ada agreed that women "actually judge men on personality, not just looks. Are you nice? Yeah I'm nice; I'll be friends with you. [For boys evaluating] a girl, it is like oh my god you're fat, and I don't like you." Sarah explained, "Guys are more focused on a girl's body while girls are more focused on everything, all aspects. A guy could be not that cute, but he could be that much cuter if he's nicer." The female campers recognized the dating double standard in that overweight males could compensate for their bodies by having nice personalities, whereas girls were strictly assessed by their bodies.

These patterns also played out in terms of how appearance influenced romantic pairings in high school. Sarah said, "For a girl, it's much harder. It's like, well, if you're an overweight girl dating an in-shape guy, it's awkward. When it does happen, people are like, 'What?' There's that, but if an overweight guy dates a girl who is in shape it's no big deal." Whereas girls could date larger boys without harsh judgment from peers, the reverse was not true. Sharon noted that romantic pairings were based on looks and "you don't usually get hot guys and ugly girls [dating each other]. Usually when you see guys with unattractive girls and they're hot, they usually don't have that many friends. . . . There's a group of guys at my school and they always go for the really hot girls because they are afraid of what their friends will say." Friendship groups served as a status control mechanism. Sharon explained the pairing of attractive boys with unattractive girls by claiming that the attractive boy was unpopular with few friends. Otherwise, boys, especially if they were high status, feared the judgment of their friends.

On the other hand, Sharon believed that girls were more supportive of each other's dating choices. Kelly said, "The guys, especially the guys in our school, it's how you look and how beautiful you are, and it depends which clique you're from. Certain guys could like you, but they wouldn't do anything about it if you don't belong to their opposite girl clique. There's like the girl version, the guy version [of cliques], and they all kind of match up." Kelly observed that people were prevented from pairing outside of their clique even if the person liked someone from a different group. Peer groups regulated who could date whom, serving as gatekeepers and a status-sorting mechanism.

Ray believed that popular girls were just as biased. He said, "I have so many girls who are popular that I know who talk to me on Facebook and ask for my advice, and they don't like their meathead of a boyfriend because he's a complete jerk to them. And I tell them to find a right guy for them. He doesn't have to be that popular quarterback of the football team to make you happy, but those girls keep going with that sort of thing. It's like they are narrow-minded in relationship categories, and it frustrates me to no end." Ray felt that he was penalized for his weight in the dating world. He said, "I'd hit it off better with the ladies if I were smaller. I'm sorry, I am 16 and I have only had one girlfriend." He said that different cliques had different standards. He explained: "The preppies judge me. My girlfriend, my last, she was in band with me. My girlfriend, all due respect, she wasn't exactly thin. She was really awesome hanging out. We could just be ourselves with each other. We didn't mind who we were. We were comfortable. She was just like me, I guess. I mean, I don't really mind, I am not in it for looks or anything. I mean, if she's quality then I really don't care what other people will say. I will be happy with who I am with." I asked him what other people said about his ex-girlfriend, and he revealed, "One time a guy made a judgmental comment about my girlfriend while I was dating her. He said she was fat and really not that pretty, and I was just ready to punch him. I told him off. But I didn't punch him because I didn't want to risk getting in trouble."

Even though Ray and his girlfriend were matched in terms of body size, other boys at school denigrated his girlfriend's looks. Whereas the popular girls at his school chose "meatheads," muscular boys who had unappealing personalities, he evaluated his girlfriend based on her positive attributes, not her physical appearance. Rather than gaining social status through his romantic relationship, Ray had to defend himself against other males who judged his girlfriend as fat and unattractive. Zach also compared himself to other boys at school and felt jealous when he saw the skinny guys hanging out with a bunch of girls. Yet he also noted that most boys who have a bunch of girlfriends are "kind of douchebags." He explained that douchebags wear Axe body spray, wear Tap Out, and shop at Abercrombie & Fitch.

While the male campers recognized that girls were often evaluated based on looks, they emphasized the importance of personality over appearance. Tom said, "I have a lot of girl friends that are bigger, and they want to lose weight to look nicer and I told them it's really how your personality is. It's all about your personality. If you have a great personality and you're big, sometimes it's better than if you had a bad personality and you were skinny. Everybody would call you the brat." Based on their own experiences with body weight, male campers were more accepting of heavier females and provided reassuring feedback to girls who wanted to lose weight. Mandy recognized this cross-gender empathy and found it comforting that there were boys at camp who struggled with their weight. She said, "There are really only like three overweight guys in 6th grade. It's nice to know that they [the boys at camp] accept you, and they're really nice about everything." At school, the girls perceived attractiveness standards as being set by high-status peers. The male campers were overall quite heavy, which led them to also feel excluded and devalued in the dating markets. By not meeting the hegemonic prescription of adolescent male body standards, the male campers adopted a perspective closer to the girls who valued personality instead of or alongside appearance considerations.

Embodied inequality structured the romantic options that adolescents had. Dating somebody who was high status meant dating a thin person, whereas dating someone overweight could potentially jeopardize one's social standing. While general popularity was intertwined with social class, dating desirability was highly gendered. The girls felt like they were evaluated based on their body size and that boys, especially high status boys, would not date heavier girls for fear of negative peer feedback. While girls characterized themselves as more accepting of boys' physical appearance, the male campers expressed acceptance of heavier girls and felt like they were also disadvantaged compared to the skinny or muscular boys who were more popular with the girls at their schools.

Discussion

Social comparisons were critical to the young people at camp problematizing their bodies. Popularity at school and peer acceptance were based on looks and social class. These body status hierarchies persist in adulthood and are often tied to social class. The girls spoke about how thin bodies were read as upper class and fat bodies were read as poor or lower class. Not only does the social status system mimic what happens in adulthood with obese adults being discriminated against, but it also leads to the internalization of this devaluation.

Being harassed by others shaped the interior life of the individual in ways that produced feelings of shame, unworthiness, and lack of confidence. The judgment and discrimination based on body size become internalized in childhood. The impact of this mistreatment is likely to be far reaching as their lack of confidence may make them feel that they do not deserve to be treated fairly in other areas of life, such as on the job market. Research has shown that the obesity stigma lingers even if weight loss occurs, which means that the damaging effects of mistreatment on a child's self-concept may persist regardless of the child's future body size.[26]

Being stigmatized and internalizing embodied inequality as a child are likely to be deeply felt because a child's self-concept is fragile, and the foundations of identity and self-esteem are being formed. Rejection and the recognition of being viewed as low status at such a young age may set people up for long-term disadvantage. In order to overcome the past, people will have to do an enormous amount of work to reframe and reclaim what was lost in childhood.

Another important implication of these findings is how deeply ingrained antifat sentiment is in our culture. Children may be unpopular or socially rejected for a number of reasons unrelated to weight. So what is different about weight? One of the earliest slurs that children use against each other is "fat." Being called fat is so loaded with negative meaning that children interpret it as one of the worst put-downs that they could get. Name calling is a form of social control and regulation and an exclusion tactic. Rather than being a neutral description, like brown-haired or tall, "fat" is an insult used to display power and perpetuate the social status system. The fat body is read as deserving to be punished and excluded even at very young ages. The fact that fatness is tied to morality and personal responsibility can lead children to think that they not only have problem bodies but also problem selves. They know that their bodies are judged negatively, and it has very real consequences in the way people treat them.

To be bullied and to hate oneself because of one's body size completely defies popular notions of childhood as a carefree time of playing and building friendships that will develop children's interactional styles and help them to form their identities. As children age into middle school, they are typically expected to begin forming an interest in dating. When children are excluded due to their weight, they are not only the victims of pain and mistreatment, but they also miss out on what is socially expected for a normal childhood based on social interactions with peers. The most heartbreaking stories were those told by campers who were bullied and harassed. The children's experiences ranged from feeling self-conscious without direct comments regarding their weight to overt, consistent victimization. Most of the campers who were bullied had social challenges that were not weight related, although most of the teasing was weight based.

The two gender-related status beliefs show how broader culture infiltrates their lives and sets up the basis for social comparisons. When they compared the clothing that thinner people wore and found that they could not wear those styles or sizes, the girls found a readily observable criterion by which to prove that their bodies were different and therefore a problem. For boys, athletics also provided a measurable outcome by which they fell short. However, some boys still regarded themselves as potentially athletic due to football players who could be heavy yet still athletic. By contrast, the girls did not ever talk about plus-sized fashion models or female celebrities with larger bodies as potential role models.

One of the primary ways that the children self-problematized was in relation to their peers. Later in the book, I will also talk about feedback from family members and medical professionals that also led some of the campers to self-problematize. Given the strong emphasis that children placed on popularity and bullying, social comparisons with peers were the primary mechanism by which children self-problematized their bodies. Children care deeply about what their peers think and suffer tremendously when they do not feel accepted. The desire to lose weight to gain social acceptance was one of the primary motivating factors for the children to attend a weight loss camp. In the next chapter, I look more closely at how the children decided to attend Camp Odyssey as a stigma-management strategy.

4

"It's Not a Fat Camp"

The Decision to Attend Camp

Sarah was a conventionally pretty 16-year-old girl with blond hair and blue eyes. At the start of camp, she was 5′7″ and weighed 171 pounds. In order to be in the normal BMI range, she would need to lose about 12 pounds. Although her family was middle class, they lived in an affluent suburb where there was pressure to achieve and to maintain a certain appearance. Known as being quiet and studious at school, Sarah was "toward the top in the middle" in terms of popularity and was never bullied or teased. However, she felt self-conscious about her body, and her mother was "cornering" her to lose the weight she had gained over the past two years. Not knowing what to do, Sarah asked her parents to send her to camp. She said that she wanted to lose weight because it would mean, "Less stress. Right now, it's like, oh my god, I don't like how I feel or look. It's frustrating." If she lost weight, she said "[I would] be more positive about myself. I would probably be more outgoing because I wouldn't be so self-conscious all the time." Given the competitive social environment at school, Sarah sought confidence and the approval of her mother through weight loss and tried to live up to expectations to be the "perfect" girl while taking Advanced Placement classes and dealing with a social environment of snobby girls at school.

Janet was a 14-year-old girl who had struggled with obesity since early childhood. At the beginning of camp, she was too heavy to be weighed using the standard scale. Given estimates from a recent doctor's visit, she weighed approximately 421 pounds. In order to be in the normal BMI range, she would have to lose 270 pounds. Her family struggled financially, and her mother was hospitalized in a nursing home for obesity-related complications. Suffering from depression, Janet was socially isolated at school. Janet wanted to attend camp due to health concerns and because it was a supportive social environment where she could be more outgoing and have fun.

Janet and Sarah were at the extreme ends of the range of people who attended the camp. Their stories illustrate the wide variety of body sizes and experiences that are encompassed in labeling children overweight. Janet's obesity was hyperstigmatized and created serious problems for her health, mobility, and social life. On the other hand, Sarah's barely overweight body did not create those hindrances, yet Sarah's weight was important to her because it conflicted with her desired social status at school and in her community. The one area that both Janet and Sarah agreed upon was that camp would influence their personalities and make them more outgoing. However, Sarah saw camp as a means to an end. She would be more outgoing after she lost weight and returned to her former life. Janet saw camp as *the* place where she could be more outgoing before returning to being isolated in her former life.

At the weight loss camp, all the children wanted to lose or manage their weight. However, not all the children had the same amount of weight to lose. Although BMI is the dominant tool of the medical profession to categorize weight, the wide range of body types and subjective perceptions complicates defining someone as overweight. Many people who appear to have a normal or muscular body composition would be categorized as overweight or even obese according to BMI measures. Therefore, it is important to point out that the children's embodied experience and approach to stigma management differed based on how they and others viewed their bodies rather than an "objective" definition of weight categorization.

In this chapter, I examine the processes by which the children engaged in stigma management related both to their weight and to their participation in a camp. Specifically, I look at how the children decided to attend a weight loss camp, how their families participated in this decision, and whether they told their peers about the camp. This chapter also describes how children negotiated the potential stigma of attending camp by constructing various definitions of the camp, ranging from a fat camp to a fitness camp, and how they determined who "really" belonged at a weight loss camp given differences in body sizes among the campers.

Family Involvement: Failed Weight Loss Attempts

Many families attempted to change their eating habits prior to enrolling their child at camp. Almost all the children tried to lose weight with family members, and many of their parents were actively dieting. However, previous attempts at changing eating habits were often short-lived and met with limited success. Melissa and her mother joined a gym, but "it's the amount of food that you put into your body instead of exercising because I didn't get any results. I just can't lose weight. It's so hard." Kyra and her mother shared a personal trainer and often went on diets together, but they usually only stayed on them for a week. Mandy's mother joined Weight Watchers and invited her to come along to learn about weight loss. Faith's mother was always dieting and often skipped breakfast in order to lose weight. Charlie and his parents tried the paleo diet.

Even when a parent was a good role model, their tactics could seem unappealing. Jenny's mother lost 50 pounds with Weight Watchers, but Jenny saw it as a very strict diet. Dana compared herself to the sacrifices her mother makes to manage her weight, and said "My mom works really hard to be in good shape, and she eats like nothing. She eats salad and fish and eggs and that's it. I could do that and be in my healthy weight range like she is, but I don't want to do that. It's not fun. It's not something I would enjoy."

Quite a few campers expressed frustration with the types of food that their parents kept in the house. Some family members tried to support weight loss by hiding the junk food they bought, but it did not work. As Kyra revealed, "Sometimes, I say I'm going to eat healthy and they're like okay, we won't buy any more junk food. And my mom, sometimes she's on board, and sometimes she's not. But my grandma and my brother have a really big sweet tooth as do I. I go in the drawer, and I find boxes of cookies, and I find Hostess cupcakes. They hide them around the house. They think I don't know that they're there."

The children revealed two major problems related to their family socialization. First, children do not have financial and transportation resources to buy food on their own. They must rely on their parents' judgment about the food that is kept in the home. Second, the family group consists of people with various tastes. While the child may wish that junk food temptations were not around, siblings and other family members may desire that type of food. Negotiating these issues and dealing with defensive parents left many children feeling as though they could not lose weight in their home environment.

Some families viewed camp not only as a means to transform their child's body but also as a way to alter the family's habits upon the child's return home. Parents told their children that they wanted them to teach the rest of the family what they learned at camp. As Kelly explained, "My mom wanted me to come home from camp and teach my family everything I've learned so that our entire family can be healthy." Mandy revealed that her mother said, "Okay, I'm sending you to this camp because I want you to lose weight but when [you] come back I want you to tell me and help me lose weight." Mandy said her mom was "not going to expect me to come back like skinny skinny but she wants it to work." Likewise Ryan's grandmother supported his time at camp because "she wanted me to learn stuff and teach it to her and the rest of the family. Everyone in my family could stand to lose weight except for my brother, who stays active."

The messages that parents sent to their children indicate that they blamed weight gain on their eating habits, yet they did not know how to change. In a reversal of the way that we typically think of childhood socialization in which parents transmit meanings and behaviors to children, the parents wanted their children to socialize them and help them to change. They identified flaws in primary socialization, which led to what they perceived as their children's weight problems. These parents wanted to support their children by changing their environment and learning what they could do to help the child and themselves as well. Thus parents viewed camp as a way to resocialize the child—and then, for the child to resocialize them.

The Emotional Impact of Weight Control Attempts

While the children reported that their parents were supportive yet frustrated, a few children also received negative feedback from extended family members. Two of the younger girls recounted being insulted by their grandfathers. Sasha took leftover cake from a birthday dinner celebration but ate it as soon as she got to her grandparents' house. When her grandmother asked if any cake was left and Sasha said no, both grandparents laughed. Her grandfather said, "Dang, you're going to be 300 pounds when you grow up. I'm not trying to be mean, but that's not healthy." Sasha cried and ran out the door to her mother who was picking her up. Likewise, Jenny told me about an emotional experience when her grandfather criticized her three weeks before camp:

> I have this one favorite dress my mom bought for me, and it fit me perfectly. And then I wore it to his [my grandpa's] house, and he said, "Why do you always wear clothes that are so tight?" I mean, it puts a lot of pressure on you, and I don't wear tight clothes at all. As you can see. My sister is the one who wears skin tight clothes, and he doesn't say anything to her so it makes you feel bad. . . . If I have one thing I like and someone thinks it looks good, I'm going to wear it. And the one thing that they know I like, they shouldn't say anything about it. They can think their opinion but they don't have to say something.

When Jenny expressed that his comment hurt her feelings, her grandmother said that he is allowed to voice his opinions. Jenny cried over what her grandfather said but maintains that they still have a very good relationship. These insensitive comments by grandfathers had a strong emotional impact due both to their directness and to the fact that other family members defended their right to critique the young girls' bodies and eating habits.

Faith's weight was central to a sibling dispute in her family. Her sister told her that her parents were mad at her because they thought she had diabetes and "my sister also said that my dad hated me because I was fat. And then when I asked him that, he said no but I do have to watch my weight like everyone else has to." Faith felt sad and told her mom, who then punished her sister.

When I asked the children about their families, a few mentioned that their fathers were trying to lose weight. Yet fathers rarely came up in relation to intervening in their children's weight. The only exceptions were Sasha and Melissa. When Sasha went swimming with her dad and wore a bathing suit, she recalled that "he looks at me in disappointment, and he said, 'You really need to start losing weight.' That just kills me. He said, 'I'm not trying to hurt your feelings, but you really need to try to lose weight.'" Melissa's father told her, "You shouldn't go to camp; you should just stop eating."

While these fathers and grandfathers made direct and cruel comments about the children's bodies, mothers were the most intensively involved with their children's weight management and the decision to attend a weight loss camp. Mothers are typically viewed as responsible for feeding their family, and they face greater scrutiny for their child's body size. Many girls reported feeling pressured by their mother to lose weight. Sarah felt helpless in conversations with her mother because she did not know how to lose weight. Sarah also felt like her mother lacked empathy for her struggle. She said, "I wish my mom knew that I had no clue what to do. She kept telling me and telling me and cornering me and making me feel awkward. My god, Mom, go away. She just told me don't eat this stuff. But if I want it, and you're telling me not to eat it, I'm going to want more. I wish she knew that it was a struggle for me and that coming up to her and asking her to go to this camp was hard for me."

Some campers reported having to manage their mother's feelings despite their own frustration when their mother would point out their weight as a problem without telling them what to do about it. Melissa said that both her parents are overweight, and her mom "always tells me all these things that's not going to help me. I don't want to be rude and hurt her feelings. She's like you should eat more salad. I'm like that doesn't do anything. I need to know stuff."

Sharon told me that being badgered by her mother made her not want to eat what her mother suggested. She contrasted herself to her "health freak" mother and aligned herself more with her father.

My mom has always been really on my back about my weight and what I eat. She does that all the time. She means it in a nice way, but I don't know, it's just like the pressure of having it all the time. Don't eat this, eat that, that's bad for you. It's really annoying. It got to the point where I just want to eat what I want to eat. I don't want to listen to you anymore. She's a health freak. She works out every day and she's on this herbal magic thing. She chews on that. My dad is kind of like me. He always says he's going to lose weight, but he never does.

Ada's mother pressured her to lose weight "all the time" and had an active role in the problematization of Ada's body. Ada said that her mom would be more helpful by

comforting me when I'm sad when people call me fat. And she's like maybe you could lose a few pounds. And I'm like that's not helping. She says I'm sorry. She makes it up to me by taking me to Claire's and getting new earrings. She does it all the time and it really hurts me. [She says] "Well maybe you should lose some pounds." Sometimes she makes me cry when she does that. I say, you don't have to be so mean. You don't have to call me fat. I don't call you fat. You're just as fat as I am. We fight about it and then I just barricade my door because my lock is broken. I barricaded it and made sure she couldn't get in. I just cry in my pillow. Just so sad and she calls me and I say why do you have to do that? That's not nice. Instead of a mother–daughter relationship we have a friend–friend relationship. Sometimes, she's strict, strict. I'm like okay, what happened to us being friends?

On the other hand, Kelly wished that her parents would take a more direct role in monitoring her eating and exercise habits. Kelly said that her parents could help her out by "not buying junk food and working out and keeping me motivated. Staying positive. Not one of those things when I give up and they're done. To have them keep doing the annoying parent nag to keep me going and working out. It's hard because they judge you, but they don't say anything to you because you're their daughter." Janet also wished that she had more family support, saying "I wish that my dad would never, ever be like let's just go to McDonalds. I wish he wouldn't ever do that. Because it's so easy when I'm hungry to want to go eat something and go have a cheeseburger." She felt like she could not say that to him because he would feel bad and become defensive.

Nearly all the overweight children had overweight parents. The parents did not know how to lose weight themselves, let alone what would work for their children. Often the advice they gave to their children was rejected outright. The children sought guidance from their parents but dismissed parental advice to eat certain foods like salad. While parents critiqued their weight, they did not effectively institute a pathway for them to actually lose weight. For Sharon and Dana, whose mothers intensively followed weight loss plans, their daughters resented the lengths their mothers went to and did not want to make those changes themselves. Parents also faced a difficult choice in their parenting style. If they intervened and pointed out their child's weight, the child would feel hurt and defensive, like Ada who barricaded herself in her room when her mother told her to lose weight. Parents who brought up weight with their children were seen as annoying. Yet other children wanted their parents to take a more active role in providing structure and holding them accountable. Prior to camp, communication with family members was frequently frustrating and fraught with emotion. Both the children and their parents felt sensitive and helpless at times, which led them to uncomfortable confrontations or avoidance of the issue altogether. This conflict caused both parents and children to view a weight loss camp as a desirable alternative.

Choosing Camp Odyssey

People often ask me whether the children were forced to attend camp by their families or if they went to camp voluntarily. For fourteen of the campers, a family member initially suggested the idea to attend a weight loss camp. Two campers reported that their parents had been looking for summer camps in general and "ended up" on websites related to weight loss camps. While parents were more likely to propose the idea to their children than the reverse, most children were receptive to the idea and did not report that they had been coerced. Zach, Bridget, Faith, Ada, Melissa, and Sharon all looked at the camp's website before agreeing to attend, which suggests that their parents wanted them to be fully informed about the camp prior to making the decision to attend. Several campers had attended an open house to gain more information in the spring. Another three said that attending camp was a mutual decision between themselves and their parents. Jenny said, "I started getting bullied, and I went online searching camps because I wanted to try to find a new, different kind of camp. And then my mom searched and found this one. We read about it, and she thought it would be really good for me to come."

While none of the first-time campers reported negative feelings about going to camp during their interviews with me or displayed overt resistance at camp, a few of the returning campers recalled their reluctance the first time they attended. Janet, who was at camp for a third time, was referred to the camp by a pediatric endocrinologist. Twelve years old at the time, she was angry that her parents sent her to camp against her will. The first week she did not want to do anything, but by the second week, she had fun and wanted to come back again the following year. Likewise, Janet's brother, Ray, said he had a "why do I have to go for a month? mentality. But I ended up going and I had a pretty fun time." Sharon also "came with a really bad attitude, but I ended up really liking it, and that's why I came back the second year."

Dana, Kelly, and Sarah initiated the idea of attending summer camp to their parents after searching online for weight loss camps. When Kelly brought up Camp Odyssey to her parents, they were "really proud of me for deciding to make the choice that I wanted to come here, to make a life change. It was very positive. They were always just telling me about how this is going to change my life and how I would feel so much better after it and they'd help me through it. They were just really surprised that I came up with it—that I wanted to do it."

However, her decision to attend a weight loss camp brought mixed feedback to Kelly, reflecting different views about whether people should accept or change their body size. One of her friends told her that "it was very stupid of me to even admit and to think that . . . then when I told them that my parents were like proud of me . . . they wanted to scream at my parents. They were like, why would your parents say something like that to you? You are fine just the way you are. You do not need to go to a weight loss camp."

After hearing her friend's reaction, Kelly remembers thinking, "My parents think I'm fat. They want me to go to camp. I was like, wait a minute, why was I so excited about this? But then I was like . . . my friend just doesn't care about weight and my parents just want me to do what I want for myself. So I just tried to make it all balance and try not to put myself in a certain direction." Kelly's friend thought that attending a weight loss camp was offensive, whereas Kelly and her parents thought it would be a positive thing to do. Kelly had to negotiate these competing reactions and actively work out a way to not interpret either her parent's or her friend's supportiveness in a negative way.

Kelly's story reflects the cultural tensions regarding children. On the one hand, her friend was astonished that her parents would allow her to problematize her body as fat and seek bodily change. In this view, parents ought to be unconditionally accepting and to shelter their children from negative body image regardless of how much the child weighs. On the other hand, Kelly's parents were supporting her own proposal to lose weight and to "change her life" for the better.

It's Not a Fat Camp

From the children's perspective, they unequivocally wanted to lose weight and clearly articulated the incentives of obtaining a thinner body. Losing weight at the camp was their primary stigma-management strategy. At the same time, they had to manage the stigma attached to attending a weight loss camp by creating clear boundaries between Camp Odyssey and a stereotypical "fat camp." The camp's description and philosophy explicitly distinguished itself from a fat camp, and this proved influential in the children's decision to participate and their enthusiasm at camp. In promotional materials, the camp was described as a fitness camp where children could have fun, be active, and lose weight.

The campers rarely referred to Camp Odyssey as a fat camp, although many worried that outsiders would perceive it as such. Their objections were based on fears of stigma and the perception that fat camps were the equivalent of boot camps with harsh rules, restrictive eating, and punishing physical activity. Having experienced the word "fat" as a put-down during encounters with bullies, some of the campers were sensitive to using it in relation to the camp. Jenny rejected the fat label saying, "I don't think of myself as fat. My sister's like a double o [clothing size], and I'm not that. It's just, I don't like the word 'fat.'" Jenny knew that she was not as thin as her very thin sister, but she did not consider herself to be fat because of its negative connotations. She felt reassured when her aunt searched online for "fat camp," and Camp Odyssey did not come up in the results. After looking at the website, Jenny determined that "it's not a fat camp. It's more of a weight management camp." Ada and her mother also used Internet search engines to determine precisely what type of camp it was. Ada said, "My mom Googled and researched a fitness camp. Camp Weight Loss was #1 and Camp Odyssey was #2. She did it again and put a different search to see if it came up the same so she put something like 'fat farm for kids.' I thought that was pretty mean. That's not going to make me want to go anymore. Something else was first. She went back to weight loss camp for kids and had a bunch of other ones and Odyssey was the fifth. And we searched weight loss management and Odyssey was first."

By using different search terms, including the stigmatizing "fat farm for kids," Ada and her mother assessed whether the camp was associated with fitness and weight management, or had a harsher, more negative view of body size. If Odyssey had come up in the search results under "fat farm" or "fat camp," Jenny and Ada said that they would have lost interest in attending.

Sharon resented her parents for sending her to what she initially perceived as a fat camp where "they were going to make us run on the treadmill for like two hours and be really mean to us and not let us eat anything. I thought it was going to be like that [television] show, *The Biggest Loser*. I didn't think the people would be nice and encouraging." After experiencing camp, she said, "It's not a regular fat camp. It's kind of like a sports camp, but I feel more comfortable because everyone is the same way." Referring to the camp as a weight loss or fitness camp made it seem less fat-shaming, and it also alleviated fears that the camp would use harsh procedures to force weight loss. The tactics that children associated with a fat camp included "constant working out," "eating gray mush of protein," "only eating salad," and "not eating that much, just feeding you like a dog."

The campers were happy that Camp Odyssey did not use those tactics. Janet described camp as "not like weight loss boot camp. It's not. I mean, you're going to lose weight while you're here because you are so much more active than you are in your regular life. The vast majority of people are anyway. You're eating better-quality food and less of it. It's about what you learn about having a healthy lifestyle in general. It's not unmanageable changes. It's teaching you how to live in the real world, as the real world is working now which is geared toward unhealthy living." Overall, the campers consistently endorsed Camp Odyssey's views on fitness and eating, although they sometimes expressed doubts about whether these lessons could be transferred to their home environment.

The Decision to Tell Others about Camp

Despite their efforts to distance Camp Odyssey from the fat camp label and their lived experience that it was not a boot camp, the specter of being stigmatized for attending a weight loss camp lingered. Melissa was embarrassed to tell her peers about camp because, "They'd be like, 'Oh you're going to a fat camp.' And I'd be like, 'No, it's a nutritional camp.' I was in an all girls class. . . . The girls are rude and obnoxious. . . . [If] I would say it is a nutritional weight loss camp then they would just turn it upside down and make it worse." Even though Melissa viewed it as a camp centered on nutrition and healthy eating, she was aware that her peers would only see it as a fat camp. She anticipated that her attempt to relabel it as a nutritional camp would be twisted and make her an even greater target for teasing. Melissa only imagined how the girls in her class would negatively interpret the weight loss camp, but Sharon actually faced a backlash the first time she attended camp: "A couple of my friends went around and told people that I was going to a fat camp. I described it to them and said it's more like a sports camp. It really is. . . . I pretty much told them that it was an athletic camp. But people stereotype people who go to weight loss camp and make them seem like losers. I came back from camp and found out everyone knew about it, and [they] were making fun of me."

While the campers insisted on using alternatives to the "fat camp" label, they knew that other people would not believe that it was a "nutritional camp" or a "sports/athletic camp." Thus the child was doubly vulnerable to insults: first by attending a camp and second for trying to cover it up. Aware of these repercussions, many campers chose to conceal their involvement with the camp. Whereas obesity is a discredited stigma, attending a weight loss camp is discreditable, and the campers could manage information about their participation.

Despite attending Camp Odyssey during the previous five summers, Dana refused to tell any of her peers. Her reluctance to talk about camp even extended to her family. She said, "We don't talk about it at my house. Everyone realizes that I go to a weight management camp every summer and have been for six years, but we don't acknowledge it. When other people ask what kind of camp I'm going to my mom will ask me if it's okay for me to tell them. But I don't tell my friends. I don't tell people." Her rationale for keeping it a secret was that she did not want to draw attention to her body size. Dana said, "Girls are always pointing out, oh I'm so fat. But I've always been under the impression that if I don't say anything, they won't notice. Why say 'Hey look at this. I'm really fat. Do you want to talk about it?' and they'll be like, 'Oh you are, aren't you?' By saying nothing, they just won't notice." Dana's strategy of avoidance was rooted in her self-consciousness about weight. The acknowledgment of attending a weight loss camp would put the spotlight on her body weight, which Dana preferred not to directly address with others.

Kyra had the opposite attitude and was nonchalant about telling others because in her view weight was visible and would inevitably be noticed by others. She told her friends she was attending the camp and "they didn't really care. They were like, 'Okay, write me a letter.'" She explained, "They can see that I'm overweight. I guess I don't really care if they know that I'm coming to this camp." The younger campers were also less likely to hide their participation from others. The few younger ones who did not tell anyone said it was simply because they did not see their friends from school over the summer and therefore did not have the opportunity to tell them.

Most of the older campers chose to tell their friends selectively. Sarah told some people that she was attending a camp but would not give its name or say that it was for weight loss because "some are just like into gossip and where I live you don't want to be gossiped. . . . so I just told my friends who I knew weren't going to say anything. I know some people won't purposely say it but it'll just come out of them. I told the people I knew wouldn't say a word." Mandy had a similar strategy. She said, "I told a couple of them that I was going to camp but I only told a few of them that I could trust that I was going to lose weight. I tell people things a lot and I know who can keep it secret and who can't. I told the people who can keep it a secret and if anyone else asks, 'Oh have you lost weight?' I'll just say yes." While they told people that they were attending a summer camp, Sarah and Mandy only revealed to a few people they trusted that it was for weight loss. Based on previous experience, they knew who would keep their participation a secret from those who would likely judge and stigmatize them. Mandy went so far as to say that she would acknowledge her weight loss without telling people where or how she lost the weight.

The campers generally feared gossip and being teased. Jenny believed that "some people would take it as a joke," and Zach said that others would "probably laugh" at him. Ada feared that she would be ridiculed for needing help to lose weight. She said that her peers would "say mean stuff like, 'Oh my god, you can't just like lose it here? Are you that stupid?'" Kelly worried about the stigma attached to attending a fat camp and the scrutiny of gaining the weight back. She explained, "It would change their view on me as that's the girl who went to fat camp for the summer. I really don't want people knowing because if it doesn't stick and if I lose a lot of weight, and then school starts and I'm happy with it, but then . . . I gain it all back. It would start a bunch more talk."

Based on the way the campers controlled information about attending Camp Odyssey, it is clear that they had a sophisticated perception of how others would view their participation in a weight loss program and that they wanted to avoid being stigmatized. Attending a weight loss camp, the very strategy that they were using to eliminate the bodily stigma of fatness, could prove stigmatizing in itself. These young people had to manage both the stigma of body weight and the stigma of camp attendance. Even if the camp produced the results they wanted, their reputation could be damaged because of the method they used to attain the result. Additionally, as Kelly points out, successful weight loss could be positively received, but subsequent weight gain would only provide more fodder for critique and judgment. The campers were in a precarious position wherein the camp could destigmatize them through weight loss, stigmatize them through participation, and then restigmatize them when they gained weight back at home.

Who Belongs at Camp?

Thus far, I have focused on how the young people who attended Camp Odyssey decided to attend a weight loss camp based on interactions with their friends, peers, and family prior to camp. While their lives "back home" influenced the campers and many conversations at camp revolved around their "real lives," the camp was a social world unto itself and a microculture that both reflected and challenged the meanings of body weight and stigma in the broader culture.

The fact that the campers themselves varied in how much they weighed created an opportunity for the campers to assess the meaning of body size within the context of the weight loss camp. Using BMI measurements taken at the beginning of camp, two campers had a normal BMI, eight were overweight, and fourteen were obese. Given the range of body sizes, the campers had to negotiate the question of who "really" belonged at a weight loss camp. Sarah said, "When I was getting ready for the [camp] dance, the other girls were like, 'I don't think you should even be here.' I'm like, 'Well, for me, I need to be here.' [They said] 'But you don't look like you're overweight.' Well, for me, I am." Sarah defended her presence at camp by citing her own subjective definition of what an appropriate body weight was for herself despite the other girls telling her that she did not appear to be overweight. In Sarah's own view of her body, her weight impacted her everyday life, her happiness, and her sense of self-worth.

When I asked Janet, the heaviest person at camp, what she thought of Sarah and the other campers who were only slightly overweight, she gave the following response:

> Some people, it's like, you are just fine. You can chill out a little bit. They're okay. I don't think they are so unhealthily overweight. Of course, there are some people who are legitimately overweight. I'm legitimately overweight. Quite a few people are legitimately overweight and need to lose weight to be

healthier. . . . [But] I don't think there's anything wrong with wanting to live a healthy lifestyle. I'm not going to say, "Get the hell out of fat camp. You're not fat." Some of the guys are bigger but not really that fat. I guess they are, not like Sarah, who really wasn't at all.

Janet defined being "legitimately overweight" as something that adversely affects one's health, and she put herself in that category. While pointing out that some people at camp did not need to be as concerned about their weight as she was, she refused to police who should attend a weight loss camp. Here, Janet referred to fat camp in a joking way ("Get the hell out of fat camp. You're not fat"), but it also underscores the idea that Camp Odyssey was not a fat camp. If it were a fat camp, then only fat people would be allowed there. Instead, the shared pursuit of weight management and health was so valued that it diminished gatekeeping due to actual body size, even in light of substantial differences such as those between Janet and Sarah.

This sentiment was shared by all the campers, who made a point to be inclusive and supportive of one another. A number of campers declared that being around other people who were trying to lose weight was the best part of camp. Mandy said, "I used to think that there were only a couple people like this and actually trying to do stuff about this but then like I see Ada and Jenny and Faith and even Hanna—she's not even that overweight but she's trying to stop it from happening." The willingness to attend a weight loss camp in itself was enough to provide a sense of rapport and to legitimize everyone there as someone who shared concerns about their body weight and had self-problematized.

Discussion

Why would a child decide to go to a weight loss camp? Were the children forced to attend by their parents? People often assume that weight loss camps are a form of punishment, and only cruel parents would send their children to a camp that forces them to lose weight. From the children's reports, parents viewed their weight as a problem, yet they did not know how to fix the problem. They felt helpless and frustrated. The children wanted guidance and structure, yet also rebelled when the parents gave advice. Under these conditions, the parents found an outside intervention to be appealing. The camp provided the environmental control and discipline that the parents could not or would not. Many of the parents struggled to lose weight themselves and viewed the camp as an organization that had the answers that would help their children. The parents then wanted their children to come home and inform them about the camp's teachings so that they could all make changes and lose weight.

Under the most generous interpretation, these parents were well intentioned and aware of their limitations. They knew that they were unable to help their children lose weight, and so they sought outside help. For parents whose children were bullied, their suffering provoked a powerful protective response that led them to send their child to a weight loss camp to improve their quality of life. Many of the children at the weight loss camp suffered tremendously due to their weight, and this is why some parents sought a solution to the problems their children faced. The parents were not trying to punish or shame their children for their weight, but they were trying to find a solution that would make their children's lives better. This is not to say that the weight loss camp itself did not have problematic components, which I will describe in later chapters; I am merely positing that the children and their parents were motivated by painful situations in their real lives and the desire to prevent them from happening in the future.

In a more critical vein, these parents outsourced their responsibility, put the burden of changing the family's habits on a child, and expected the camp to solve a problem that they could not. If the parents could not lose weight, how did they expect their children to be able to? Instead of putting the responsibility on the children or the camp, the parents could have made changes in their family's lifestyle rather than waiting for the child to come back from camp to teach them new habits. Alternatively, families could have just outright accepted their child's body.

In addition to the burdensome expectations that the children had to manage, they also had to negotiate the potential stigma of attending a weight loss camp. While they wanted to lose weight to gain peer acceptance, they did not want their peers to know that it was through a weight loss camp. The children used careful language to distance Camp Odyssey from a fat camp, and they selectively managed the information to prevent untrustworthy friends from gossiping about them, which could undermine their already precarious reputation.

Each of the children and their families made the decision to enroll in a weight loss camp. Each child viewed their body as a problem and wanted to lose weight. Yet, once they got to camp, there was a wide variety of body sizes and different amounts of weight that they wanted to lose. The naming and framing of the camp as something other than a fat camp also opened the doors to allowing campers who were not significantly overweight or had normal BMIs. While the children noted these body size differences, they endorsed the notion that the camp was based on fitness or weight management because it protected their own self-image and aided in stigma management. If the camp's purpose was for children to become healthier, rather than being a fat camp, participants did not have to be fat to attend. This meant that no one was going to be rejected for being too thin. A child with a normal BMI or one who was only slightly overweight could attend under the rationale that this person wanted to prevent weight gain from occurring. Living amid a culture of fat phobia, even a thin or normal body is under threat of fatness; therefore, weight intervention is accepted. This was certainly the case for Sarah and Jacob, siblings who had a slightly overweight and normal BMI, respectively. The desire to be thinner—the normative discontent with body size—was so prevalent that the camp directors allowed them to attend, and the other campers ultimately accepted their presence even though their bodies were not viewed as being unhealthy or as "legitimately" problematic as other bodies at camp.

5

"They Were Born Lucky"

Weight Attribution among
the Campers

It's just they're lucky. They were born lucky, and they have a good metabolism. I have a friend who eats anything she wants. I was talking to her, and she's like, "I don't understand. I eat probably twice as much food as you at breakfast and dinner and lunch, and I don't gain a thing. It's not fair for you." She eats snacks; [she] eats a whole bag of chips and doesn't gain anything.
—Mandy

One aspect of embodied inequality is the sense of microlevel injustice when people confront why they are disadvantaged while others are not. As Mandy describes, the campers recognized that it was not fair that some of their friends, siblings, and peers could engage in the same eating behaviors as they did without gaining weight. Their friends were "born lucky" because they had a metabolic system that burned calories at a faster rate. The idea that body size is something we are born with or at least set up for based on metabolism resonates because of the observable variety in eating habits and body weight outcomes. Causal attributions also have important stakes for how individuals view their own body projects based on cultural beliefs that make body weight a matter of personal responsibility. To say that body size is solely the result of a metabolic lottery renders the dieting industry useless, and the person who wants to reshape her body hopeless. If weight is ultimately the outcome of a predetermined metabolic structure, then what can the "unlucky" possibly do to become thin?

Unsurprisingly, the Camp Odyssey program did not endorse the view that weight is a matter of luck or predestined at birth. They wanted the campers to believe that they could lose weight through effort. However, the directors and counselors had to negotiate the fact that the campers, in their lived experience, saw differences in body size as a matter of injustice and luck because other people in their lives did not have to exert the extraordinary effort that the camp asked of them. In this chapter, I explore the tensions and contradictions in the causal attributions used at camp. I explain how the campers viewed the sources of their weight gain and how the camp attempted to convince them to adopt certain attributions and to reject others.

Attribution

Attribution involves how people explain the causes of their own or others' behaviors and provides insight into how people view the amount of control they have over their lives.[1] Behavior is influenced by a person's locus of control, which is connected to emotion, especially self-esteem.[2] Bernard Weiner's attribution theory is based on internal versus external locus of control, the stability of the cause, and whether the condition is controllable or uncontrollable. The interaction of these three elements results in varying emotions, motivation, and behaviors. I extend Weiner's attribution theory to how children at a weight loss camp viewed the causes of their weight and their own personal stake in changing their bodies. I will particularly focus on the four dimensions of causality that Weiner describes: ability, effort, task difficulty, and luck.

Ability is a dimension of causality that is internal, stable, and not controllable. Lack of ability means that there is something inherent within that makes losing weight impossible. Applying this to body size, the ability to be thin is seen as coming from within, unlikely to change in the future, and unable to be controlled by the person. This attribution suggests that body size is deterministic, inherent, and natural. Internal uncontrollable causes of failure are associated with feelings of shame and humiliation, and stable causes lead to hopelessness. Therefore, those campers who attribute their weight to a lack of ability to lose weight are expected to have lower self-esteem.

Like ability, effort comes from within, yet it is subject to change and controllable by the person. If failure is attributed to low effort, people tend to expect a different, more successful outcome when effort is increased. People feel pride when they succeed due to effort because it comes from an internal source. However, failure due to an internal, controllable cause, such as lack of effort, can also lead to guilt and regret. Thus campers who attribute their weight to a lack of effort will likely have low self-esteem but maintain hope that they will be able to change in the future.

Task difficulty, on the other hand, deals with the perceived difficulty of the task. Viewing a task as highly difficult signifies that weight loss is unlikely to be achieved. Weiner states that task difficulty is external, stable, and uncontrollable, although sometimes controllable by others. For example, the student cannot control the difficulty of the test so it is external to the student; however, a teacher has the control to make an exam easier in the future. There is no guarantee that the teacher will do so, and task difficulty may simply be uncontrollable by anyone. In terms of body weight, if campers view weight loss to be difficult due to stable, external factors, they will likely feel hopeless and expect future failure. However, campers who view weight loss as extremely difficult and yet still lose weight will feel pride. Task difficulty can affect self-esteem in two ways, depending on the outcome: success leads to pride, and failure leads to hopelessness. Both ability and task difficulty are stable and not controllable.

The final dimension of causality is when an outcome is attributed to luck, which is external, unstable, and uncontrollable. If an outcome is caused by luck, the person cannot take responsibility for success so pride is lower. In terms of body weight, luck would mean that a person is thin or loses weight without effort. Luck is subject to future change, so hope can be maintained. In a reversal of Weiner's formulation, luck could run out since it is unstable. Luck may also be linked to magical thinking (i.e., "someday I will lose weight and feel great about myself").

Further, people may sometimes hold beliefs and ideas that contradict the attributions that they use for themselves. In this case, the children made a distinction between the attributions of weight for "some people" or "other people" versus the explanations that they gave for why they personally were overweight. Regardless of how the campers viewed the causes of weight gain, the camp attempted to socialize the children to adopt their preferred attribution, that body weight is a result of effort, and to reject other possible explanations.

This exchange with Sarah shows the multiple attributions she made and how they traversed the various causal dimensions.

SARAH: I think some people aren't [overweight] because they take care of themselves or they just have a high metabolism. Some people aren't [thin] because it could be medical. They just can't, they're just overweight, and there is nothing they can do. They can always do something, but they're. . . .

And some people just don't take care of themselves. And some people may not be overweight at first and not realize they aren't taking care of themselves and [their] habits catch up.

LB: The not taking care of yourself thing, what does that mean to you?

SARAH: You're not eating healthy foods. There's no bad foods, but you're eating too much of the high in fat foods and high calories. You're just focusing on eating right, but you're not exercising or you're just focusing on exercising but not eating right. You have to have both.

LB: The whole package.

SARAH: If you are in shape, you are taking care of everything. You're doing both.

First, Sarah offered two explanations for thinness: either people "take care of themselves" or they *just* have a high metabolism. According to Sarah, taking care of yourself means eating healthy foods and exercising. The attribution of taking care of yourself is effort based. On the other hand, she gave the explanation that some people are thin without making any effort because they simply have a high metabolism. This falls under the luck attribution because their metabolism is something that was bestowed upon them with no effort, but it is unstable because their luck could run out. She later says that people who are not taking care of themselves risk becoming overweight because their habits of not eating healthy foods and exercising enough may catch up to them. Thus the only surefire way to be thin is through effort. As I will explain later in this chapter, Sarah's explanations for thinness mapped perfectly onto the camp's messages about weight management, effort, and the untrustworthiness of a lucky metabolism. In fact, her words about taking care of yourself and habits can be traced almost verbatim to Fay's lectures during Education sessions.

However, when addressing why some people are overweight, Sarah allowed for a medical explanation of obesity that defied the camp's messages. Sarah said, "They just can't, they're just overweight, and there is nothing they can do. They can always do something, but they're. . . ." Sarah's medical attribution speaks to the causal dimension of ability, and that some people may lack the ability to lose weight. She said that they "just can't" and "there is nothing they can do." This means that no amount of effort will change their body because an underlying medical condition overpowers their body's ability to lose weight and be thin.

Yet Sarah immediately backtracked after making such a powerful, deterministic statement and said, "They can always do something, but they're . . ." without finishing the sentence. I do not know how Sarah would have completed her thought, but I can speculate that she was making the point that people with medical conditions can "always do something" and make an effort, but they are still going to be overweight. In the next sentence, she contrasted this group of people who are medically fated to be overweight to how "some people" are overweight due to not taking care of themselves. Sarah's definition of taking care of yourself indicates not only the enormous amount of effort involved in weight management, but it also points to the causality dimension of task difficulty in that it is not enough to only monitor food intake or only exercise, but that people who successfully take care of themselves do both.

Genetic and Biological Explanations

Like Sarah, some of the other campers surmised that obesity could be caused by biological and genetic factors. However, these underlying causes did not map neatly onto just one type of attribution. Rather, they could be invoked in relation to multiple types of attributions, in conjunction with other explanations, or as part of a complex narrative that bridged attributions.

None of the campers said that a genetic, medical, metabolic, or biological explanation was the *sole* reason why some people were overweight and others were not. Further, none of the campers said that the reason why they personally were overweight was entirely due to a biological cause. Instead, they brought up genetics as one possible explanation among several. Some people said that biology was an underlying cause that could hinder one's ability to lose weight but that improving habits could keep it under control, whereas others were more deterministic.

As with Sarah's explanations for body weight, medical reasons were often given alongside habits and effort. Jenny said, "I think some are overweight because maybe they don't care. Maybe they have, I've heard of problems with your weight because you can't like, your brain says you're hungry when your stomach says you are full. They could have health problems." Like Sarah's contrast to people who don't take care of themselves, Jenny brings up people who don't care and then references a medical condition, most likely a genetic disorder like Prader–Willi syndrome, which causes an insatiable appetite but is exceptionally rare in the population. Jenny also later said that "maybe skinny people do watch their weight and make sure they're eating right."

The most common way that the campers talked about genetics, though, was in reference to their own families. Tom said, "It definitely has to do with your history, your family history. The way you were genetically made." Kyra alluded to within-family genetic diversity, "I think a lot of it has to do with genes. Some people have a skinny brother or sister. Like most of the people in my family are average sized." Kyra explained that some siblings may inherit "thin" genes, which allows them to be "skinny" or average sized whereas other children are genetically set up to gain weight.

Dana explained that her weight was related to her family's genes. She said, "I'm overweight because my whole family is. It's hereditary." In her view, she and her family had to resist a "normal" lifestyle in order to combat their genes. Dana could not understand "why there are other people who can be totally inactive and eat a lot and still be in shape and why we can't. . . . Me and my family, we just did what normal people do, and we didn't go to the gym every day or eat salad for every meal. That's not what normal people do, so we can't be like normal people. It's a big deal. Everyone who is overweight, you can't be like a normal person. You have to do different things, and it's not fun."

Dana's account bridges the attributions of ability, effort, and task difficulty. She believed that she lacked the genetic ability to be effortlessly thin. Instead, losing weight was extremely difficult and required drastic behavioral changes and effort to even potentially overcome her genetic makeup. The external aspect of task difficulty was illuminated by her examples of the "normal" lifestyle that she would have to forgo, such as not having to work out every day or not eating salads for meals.

Attributing body weight to ability was in direct opposition to how the camp wanted children to view weight loss. Lacking the ability to control weight meant that the body was unlikely to change over time, and it was not controllable by the individual. The camp did not want the children to believe that they could not control their weight and that they were destined to be overweight for life. Therefore, they attempted to defuse the ability attribution by reaffirming the importance of self-control. For example, the children were taught that they needed to change their thought patterns to regard weight as changeable and controllable.

During Education sessions, the children were instructed that changing one's thoughts can be intentional and learned. To demonstrate, the campers had to turn deprivation statements into satisfaction statements. For example, a statement alluding to the ability attribution is, "I've always been overweight, so I always will be." This deprivation statement renders body weight as deterministic and inherent. In order to shift this attribution from ability to effort, the campers were taught to convert the thought into a satisfaction statement that focused on individual control, such as, "I am going to start paying attention to my hunger and fullness." Satisfaction statements were intentional and positive because they centered on the idea that an overweight body was unstable. The hope of future change was funneled into tasks, such as using the hunger scale, that were touted as controllable.

The other biologically rooted attribution that consistently came up was metabolism. However, unlike genetics or medical disorders, the way campers viewed metabolism was less fixed and stable. Metabolism was seen as a matter of luck. Luck means that a person is thin or loses weight without effort. A common narrative among campers was that some people are simply lucky to be "naturally" thin due to an advantageous metabolism. Tom explained, "I have a friend who eats the same way I eat, all day, every day. Sometimes even worse than I eat. He'll eat a Pepsi, a bag of Chex Mix, and tons of food for lunch and he's maybe 5 and a half foot and 100 pounds, but he eats like he's my size. He has such a fast metabolism. He has to eat a lot because it just burns off so quick."

Kelly said that weight was either a matter of luck or habits:

> I always thought that you were born the way you were built. There's always the saying like you're big boned. Because there's just certain girls who are super tiny and I feel like if they were to just stop exercising. I don't even know if they are exercising. If they ate a ton of junk food, would they even gain weight? They are just so tiny. Other people I feel like it is their own fault because they do have McDonald's every day for every single meal, . . . It could just be like, people who aren't overweight are either really lucky or they're doing something. They realize they don't want to be overweight so they're doing something to stop it.

In this account, Kelly goes between two attributions. People who do not make an effort but remain thin are lucky, while those who make an effort did so because "they realize they don't want to be overweight." Kelly reinforced the idea that body size is a choice and controllable for those who are not lucky enough to be thin.

One of the unique features of the camp was that it was embedded in a larger summer camp that was not based on weight loss. Camp Odyssey and Camp Jay shared a cafeteria. The Odyssey campers certainly noticed the different foods being served and compared their bodies to the Jay campers. I often heard them remark about how skinny the Jay campers were and how unfair it was that they got to eat all of the "bad" foods and not gain weight. In my field notes, I could not help but make the same type of contrast: "It is so strange that Camp Jay seems to disprove everything that they are teaching at Camp Odyssey. The Jay kids scarf down their food and eat junk food. They don't eat mindfully. They don't care about portion sizes. And they really are skinny. It is frustrating and weird. Fay says that it will catch up with them someday. But why did it catch up to our kids now?"

Out of the four attributions, luck was the one that most captured the injustice felt by the campers. It was also the catchall attribution for what was most inexplicable about how body size was distributed. One day, a camper confronted Fay with the fact that some people are skinny even though they eat whatever they want. Fay responded with several refutations. First, she said, "Just remember that they won't always be that way, and it will catch up to them." This points to the fact that luck is unstable and could potentially run out. Second, Fay said, "This is a rare person, only one person compared to everyone you know. Americans are constantly struggling with their weight." Here, she suggests that those people are infrequent exceptions and the campers' experience of trying to lose weight is the normal American way. Finally, she said,

"They may not be healthy. They may not be able to run." This idea that thinness does not equal health or physical fitness was a theme throughout camp. The program directors referred to fitness as an outcome that allowed them to maneuver past the luck attribution and return to effort.

Family Habits and Lifestyle

The children identified family habits and emotional problems as contributing to weight gain and hindering efforts to lose weight. When asked why some people are overweight and others are not, Ada said, "They were raised differently. Those eating habits started at a certain age." Ada told me that an overweight godsister influenced her eating habits at a young age:

> She would visit me sometimes, and she would give me way too much. I'd see that she finished all of her food and [think] well, maybe I should finish all of mine. And then, I would do that. I would develop these eating habits, and then I would just keep eating the same McDonald's burger. Getting into the medium fries or the large fries, and then I'd eat them all myself and eat them so fast. By the time I'm done, I'd be like, ugh . . . when they go out to eat, I could get the kids burger, but they got the adult burger so I got the adult burger. And I was like, ooh I feel so stuffed and I can't even finish all my food. And they ate it, and I was like I can finish it. I was trying to be like them. My godsister moved away, but then I still had the bad eating habits.

Ada attributed her weight gain to emulating the eating habits of her godsister and following her example to order adult-sized burgers and finishing all of her food. In her recollection of these events, Ada recalls actively "trying to be like them" and being motivated to match what the adults were eating. Ada clearly narrated these "bad" eating habits through the lens of the camp's messages about overriding fullness cues, eating until you are "stuffed," having large portion sizes, and consuming fast food.

Ada focused on eating habits, whereas Ryan attributed weight gain to inactivity. While Ryan also pointed out that he modeled his behavior after an adult in his life, he viewed his indolence as a "choice" to follow his father's example. He said, "I think the difference is for some people, it's just activity. I think it comes in with the parents because most people are raised up how their parents raised them. Still, I have had the choice to make activity [part of my life], but I kind of went the lazy way. That is the way my dad is, and I was following him."

Ryan and Ada both expressed their agency in terms of making conscious decisions to follow the example of adults. They constructed a sense of shared responsibility in which the adults' bad habits were characterized as relatively neutral until the child *chose* to follow their example. However, some might object to giving the child any responsibility in this situation and argue that it is always the adult's responsibility to set boundaries and be a good role model. The child should not be put in the situation to emulate bad habits, and the adults should have intervened to force Ada to order the child-sized burger or to encourage Ryan's physical activity.

Looking back on their childhoods, both Kelly and Ray wished that their parents had taken more control of their eating and exercise habits. Kelly compared her family's habits to her friend's family. She said, "When I think about it, with my friend's family, she didn't grow up having [Little] Debbie snacks or popcorn or those types of things in her house, and so they're all very tiny. It's kind of one of those things, I'm like, wow, I wish they had watched it a little bit more and had not given us so much junk food every time we ask. . . . My dad always tells me that he wishes they kept us in sports more and started us when we were little."

According to Kelly, the choices that her parents made regarding physical activity and food led to her weight gain. If she had been raised in a different family that did not buy junk food and encouraged athletic activity, she believes that she would have been thinner like her friend. Mike reinforced the importance of parental responsibility when reflecting on his own childhood:

> I think it comes down to lifestyle and parenting. If you raise your kid to eat veggies and get active and have fun, but don't force them to do it, then you're going to probably have a really good, active kid. But if you're not going to be strict enough right away. . . . You get your kids to acquire tastes by an early age; it sets a whole life for them. It was like that for me. My mom always bought unhealthy food. She tried to get me to eat vegetables, and I hated them, and then she just never fed them to me again. All due respect to my dear old mother, she was just never firm to me in that regard. And now it shows right now.

Ray pointed to parenting style as the cause of his weight gain. He believed that if his mother had been more authoritative when it came to making him eat vegetables, he would have acquired a taste for healthy food and not gained so much weight.

While Ray cautioned against parents being overly strict and controlling, his own parents' lax attitude resulted in his eating habits, which led to weight gain at a very young age. Ray recalled only being relatively "normal" in kindergarten when he weighed 60 pounds compared to his peers who were 50 pounds. He said, "I figured, oh I'm just a little bigger than everyone else. I'm not like overly fat or anything. But I mean, by the time I was 160 pounds in 4th grade, my dad still really hadn't done much about it. I figured I was normal." Ray played football successfully because the linemen were small, and he could just push them over. As he got into middle school, though, he said, "I was building fat, not muscle. By 6th or 7th grade, I was a weakling, I was 200, 230 pounds." His parents did not start talking to him about his weight until he was in 7th or 8th grade. By his freshman year of high school, he peaked when he weighed in at 310 pounds at his winter doctor's appointment. Ray said, "I love my parents, but I wasn't really raised the right way, raised to be healthy. I was raised to be an athlete, but I was never raised about food or constant activity." Not only did his parents provide an unhealthy food environment, they did not address his weight gain until adolescence, when he began having serious health problems.

The family was a central figure looming over the camp's lessons regarding weight loss and attribution. Since the children were living away from their parents, the camp highlighted their personal autonomy. If the camp did not believe that the campers could make independent choices separate from their family's influence, then the camp would have required the families to attend camp. However, the camp implicitly believed that if an individual, even a child, could learn new habits, they could adopt those new habits and adapt them to their home environment. Thus, the camp's resocialization efforts were premised on the belief that an individual child could overpower the family's influence.

Emotional Problems

A few campers pointed out that traumatic events and emotional eating can lead to weight gain. When asked why some people are overweight, Melissa talked about deaths more generally before linking it to her personal story saying, "Probably a family member died in their family. Maybe other kids went through something that other people haven't. Somebody died or something tragic happened. My grandma passed away, and I started gaining a lot of weight. I wasn't really that big when she passed away, but I gained a lot of weight. That's why I'm this number." After Melissa's wealthy paternal grandmother died, her father's siblings disputed the will and forced Melissa's family to move out of their grandmother's house. She said, "So everything is all crazy. My family is all messed up. I'm just upset. It's just crazy."

As one of the attributions she named for why others are overweight, Jenny talked about overweight students at her school who "don't care."

LB: What do you mean that some people may not care?
JENNY: There's people in my school who I know they don't care. They don't care about their schoolwork. They don't care what they wear. They don't try at all.
LB: And they don't care about their weight?

JENNY: At lunch, they just eat, eat, eat.

LB: Does that make you think badly of them?

JENNY: No. I think there might be something else that's going on with them. Or something kind of happened that made them like that.

Jenny related overeating to not caring about schoolwork or appearance in general and believed that they acted that way due to troubled circumstances. Sharon connected emotional eating to family problems and observed, "I find that most people who are overweight have really messed up lives. Because they eat to get their feelings out. And they take their feelings out on food. I bet you most of the people here have messed up lives. . . . Most of the people with the really messed up lives have the really messed up parents whose parents don't really want to see them."

Jasmine contrasted overweight and underweight people with what she perceived as their corresponding emotional issues saying, "Well, for the overweight people it could be that they're really depressed, and food is their best friend. They really don't know how to socialize with people. And for skinny people, I think it's an anxiety problem. They probably don't eat at all or really, really small portions. Or they like throw up a lot when they get done eating." Jasmine said that overweight people emotionally eat because they are depressed and isolated, whereas thin people do not eat or eat very little because they are anxious or bulimic. When I asked her why she was overweight, she said,

I don't know why do I eat. I really don't. I really don't know. I think I do because it's probably there. It's just there, and I probably have nothing to do. It's like when I'm up in the house, and it's one of those days when you got to clean up and stuff. And then I take a break and just sit there, just get lazy on the couch. And then all of the sudden you watch a commercial and you're like instantly hungry, just like that. You just want everything, all the things that's in the refrigerator.

She did not directly refer to her own depression or isolation like she did when she spoke generally, but she attributed her eating to boredom when she was stuck in her house with nothing to do. Watching television triggered her cravings, and she recalled going to the refrigerator to eat.

Janet talked about how people are conditioned to emotionally eat. She said, "If people associate eating pot roast with being happy and with being with their family, when they're sad they're going to want some pot roast. It has a lot to do with comfort food. People who eat ice cream when they're sad. Stuff like that." Janet then reflected on her own emotional eating:

JANET: I had a massive, massive problem with when I am bored, I am sad, this sucks, let's eat.

LB: When you eat and it's emotional eating, does it make you less bored, less sad? Does it solve the problem?

JANET: There's the catch 22. You just eat. It doesn't help. Of course, it doesn't help. And then you just feel ashamed, just worse but it keeps happening. Weird.

LB: Right, then you feel worse and because you feel worse, you eat more. It's a cycle.

JANET: I have actually done that before. It's kind of, even thinking that I've even done that, I'm ashamed of that. Ugh.

Janet then likened her eating to "bulimia without vomiting. Just binge, no purge." When I asked her if the camp program had the resources or knowledge to adequately address binge eating, she replied, "I think they need to put more emphasis on that. They don't emphasize a lot of problems I've had enough. Binge eating. They don't talk about that enough. They don't do so much about emotional eating, like checking before you eat. I think they did last year, but they haven't this year at all. Before you eat, are you really hungry? Are you? And how do you feel, really? Is food really what you need now?"

I agreed with Janet's assessment that the camp program did not adequately address the emotional, disordered, and addictive aspects of eating and weight gain. In this way, Camp Odyssey was similar to other weight loss programs that emphasized education, rational decision making, and willpower over addressing the deeper emotional needs of some participants.[3] During the entire month at camp, Fay only devoted one Education session to talking about emotions. She began that session by reading the poem, "What If" by Shel Silverstein, which is a series of anxious questions that the protagonists thinks about at nighttime. Fay told the children, "Worrying at night is normal. Having what ifs is normal. There are difficult times in life. People think of childhood as a time of joy, but kids are human, too, and feel disappointment and hurt. We cannot expect perfection." Fay opened the conversation by validating the complex emotions and anxieties that children have and telling them that it is normal to have those emotions.

She then asked them how they handle it when life is tough. A few of the campers made comments related to finding moral support and talking to others about their problems. Fay encouraged them to use physical activity to release their emotions:

We want a way to channel it out. Keeping it in isn't healthy. People can use exercise when they are stressed, like power walking or using a punching bag. Do not ignore feelings of hurt and disappointment, but don't get stuck in negative feelings and complain all the time. If people get stuck in bad feelings and are sad, they can eat and eat and just get bigger. It might kill them. Emotions lead to eating habits. When you feel good, strong, satisfied, you make better decisions. It is important to stay in touch with your emotions.

Kevin said that he drinks a soda when he is depressed, and it does make him feel better. Fay cut him off to say that moving changes the biochemistry in the brain without acknowledging that food or sugary drinks can be temporarily comforting. Fay continually emphasized physical movement as the solution. She said that if they are bored, upset, or tired, they should stay away from food and find a substitute for eating. While Fay wanted the children to deal with their emotions, she refused to validate the short-term soothing that food can provide or to help the children cope with emotions in any way other than athletic output.

In Fay's view, emotions underlie eating habits and decision making. Children should not deny their emotions, but rather use the emotions to fuel physical activity rather than eating. She characterized emotional eating as being "stuck" in negativity and eating so much that they could die. This overly simplistic solution of swapping eating for physical activity made it seem like the body could overcome deep-seated emotional patterns and even mental illness by working out. While physical activity could potentially help some people feel better, it cannot substitute for the professional mental health counseling needed by people suffering from binge eating disorder, mental illness, or traumatic family situations. The camp did not offer counseling, and never provided information about the benefits of mental health treatment.

Losing Weight Is Hard

When I asked the campers why some people are overweight and others are not and why they are overweight, they did not typically answer by saying that it is because losing weight is hard to do. However, their most common answer when I asked what they wished other people knew about what it was like to be overweight was that they wished other people knew how hard it was both to be overweight and how difficult it was to lose weight.

Janet explained the challenge of weight management by referencing eating disorders. She said, "I'm sure it looks a lot simpler than it is. I'm sure it's a lot simpler to tell an anorexic person to eat a cheeseburger. It seems so easy, but it's not. It's not at all. . . . It's not easy, it's not as simple as just eat a cheeseburger or not as simple just eat more salad and take a walk." Sharon agreed, "I have friends who will talk about people who are overweight, and they'll be like, why doesn't she just do something about it? Why doesn't she just lose weight? It's really not that easy. There could be a lot more stuff going on in her life that you don't know about. It just bothers me when people say stuff like that. There's a lot more to it than what they think."

In addition to the difficulty of losing weight, the children saw other people as not understanding how long it takes to lose weight. Sarah said, "People didn't realize how much easier it is to gain weight than it is to lose it. They should be more understanding of that; stuff happens." Ada said: "You become like this, and you can't change it, and it takes forever to change. It takes like 5 seconds to become like this and an hour to get back to it, as a comparison. If you think about it, it takes five years to change this, for example, and ten minutes to get like this. It's like, well, I wasn't always like this. It just happened. Maybe I'm going to grow out of it, maybe I won't. If not, maybe I was just born like this. I was born this way." Ada contrasts the slow and arduous process of losing weight through effort compared to the ease and quickness of gaining weight. She also brings up an interesting temporal component in saying that she was not always this heavy, and "it just happened." Then she allows for the possibility that she will outgrow her weight gain. If she does not, she will come to the recognition that she was "born this way." If she does not lose weight in the future because it is too difficult, Ada will change her attribution from effort, which allows for the changeability over time, to a deterministic lack of ability in which she evokes an intrinsic "born like this" explanation. According to Ada, only time and her future body will tell whether she was born to be overweight or whether this was a temporary stage in her development.

At camp, task difficulty was regarded as simply needing a cognitive shift in attribution. Fay emphasized the power of retraining the brain and habits through learning. She told them that when people learn things easily, they equate it to natural ability, yet there are skills that can be learned by watching and practicing that will eventually feel just as natural as the easy tasks. The campers were told that the brain was a muscle that could be strengthened and that "things are hard until it is easy." In terms of weight management, Fay said, "We use good strategies, and it becomes easy." The camp staff wanted them to leave camp knowing that they could do hard things and that change came through hard work. Fay said that self-esteem is not based on other people saying nice things about you, but that feelings of self-accomplishment come from setting goals to do hard things and then doing them.

Fay described the process of changing habits as a groove. She said that the old and new ways of being are two poles at the end of a U-shaped curve. When people set out to make changes, they feel excited at first, but the middle is hard. At the bottom of the U, a person feels discouragement. They may want to quit and feel like they are never going to make it or climb out of the groove. People do not know how close they are to the end until they are really close. The end point is when the habit is established and something like eating to a 5 on the hunger scale is not a big deal. The groove analogy addressed the difficulty of weight loss. A habit is not only repeated behavior, it is also a way of being that feels natural. Making a new habit feel as natural as the old one is challenging, but, according to Camp Odyssey, it is possible. The new groove, the end point of the U-curve, referred to a way of being that feels effortless and does not require intent, internal struggle, or willpower to maintain.

The directors of Camp Odyssey thought that children could establish a new groove during their time at camp because it provided a radical environmental change. Instead of being stuck in old ways, camp could establish a new path and better habits. By taking kids out of their former environments and patterns, the camp supposedly allowed them to establish a new groove. The inherent challenge with establishing a new groove in a completely different environment from home was that the children would return to their old environment in a short time. Fay repeatedly told the children that the new groove was fragile and vulnerable, so they would have to make an enormous effort to preserve their new habits after they left camp.

Effort and the Body Project

During interviews, most of the children pointed to eating and exercise habits as being the main determinant of their own weight. Some of the campers believed that controlling body weight can occur either through exercise or eating healthy. For example, Zach said, "Well, there are two different kinds. People who eat a lot and exercise a lot. And the people who don't exercise but don't eat as much. I just like to stay in most of the day, and I don't really do stuff." Bridget said that some people are overweight based on "eating habits and exercise habits." Faith said "the skinnier people . . . have less portions of food. The overweight people have bigger portions, and they don't get as much exercise as the people who are the right number." Charlie said that it has to do with "probably because they actually do more physical activity. They go out for more sports and do a little bit more." Mandy said, "I think that I eat too much, and I don't eat slow enough. I don't get out and exercise enough because like the only sport I'm in is softball, and it meets once a week. You get pretty much three hours of exercise once a week."

Jacob connected habits and self-control. He said, "I feel some are overweight because they just eat the foods that they want. They don't really think about what they're eating. They just, if they want it, they'll just have it. And then once they probably notice that they're overweight they think, 'Oh, I shouldn't have done that.' But then like, some people are more healthy because they think about what they eat and they exercise. They balance all their meals and things like that."

Kelly talked about how a strong desire to lose weight leads to effort. She said, "I would hope that yeah, if you really want it that bad then you would do something about it. I mean my parents tell me all the time, if you want it that bad, you would have done it, blah blah blah. You would have done it yourself. You would have done something so that you could have made sure that happened." Courtney said that she encourages herself, and she believes "It can get better if I just try and try and try."

The camp directors consistently emphasized the importance of self-control. One day, Fay told them a story about when she was learning how to ski, and her companion yelled out to her, "Are you riding those skis or driving them?" Fay said this is a good way to think about every facet of life—schoolwork, hobbies, food, and exercise. She said that you can be in control or let your life be in control; you can be a spectator or actively making decisions. Then she gave examples of decisions they could make related to weight loss, such as eating part of a restaurant portion or finding seasonal sports. Finally, she said that a person who is driving his or her life is actively engaged in life. She asked them, "What kind of person do you want to be? Do you just want to slide by?"

The camp attempted to socialize its participants to attribute weight loss to effort. Specifically, they believed that children needed to use effort in order to practice self-control, which would lead to weight loss. Learning to delay gratification was seen as one of the most important factors of self-control. Early in the first week, Fay described a classic psychological research study in which 4-year-old children were put in a room with a marshmallow. The subjects were told that if they waited for the researcher to come back, they would get another marshmallow. Half ate the marshmallow and half waited. The half who waited had strategies to distract from eating the marshmallow, such as humming, playing, sitting on their hands, and not looking at it. When the researchers followed up with the "marshmallow kids" later in life, they found that those who waited did better in school, went to college, had higher-paying jobs, and were in stable, healthy relationships. Camp leaders wanted the children to internalize the idea that they could delay gratification through learned strategies and practice. Fay told them, "With weight management, we use good strategies, and it becomes easy." By framing delayed gratification as something that comes from within and that is subject to an individual's will, the camp saw its role as giving the campers the tools they would need to change their past habits of immediate gratification, which they viewed as a major culprit for weight gain.

The campers were instructed to write down specific goals related to doing things that required practice and effort. Fay shared the motivational quote, "If I always do what I've always done, I'll always get what I've always gotten." The message was that if they wanted a different outcome, they needed to challenge themselves to approach their lives in a different way. Fay said that they could learn any skill as long as they put forth the effort to practice it. They discussed strategies in six areas: eating, food, physical activity, social support, environmental cues, and self-motivation. During the last week of camp, Fay worked passionately during the Education sessions to have the campers write an individualized plan for each of the six areas. Fay referred to herself as a "barracuda" when it came to their plans. She wanted them to fill out a chart with specific and doable behaviors, and she was curt and direct if their behaviors were not specific enough. She told them, "I'm serious when kids go home and haven't practiced this muscle—they haven't learned to push the food away or move, they fail. You have to work on self-control."

Below is a sample chart from one of the campers:

ENVIRONMENT
Food out of view
Smaller plates/bowls
Grocery list/shopping
Don't buy in bulk

FOOD
Portions—hand signals
Read labels
Reduce soda (once a week)
Buy fruits and veggies, not chips

EATING
MyPlate
Mindful—chew more,
  check in with stomach
Partnering protein
Leave one bite

SUPPORT
Work out with family member
Use recipes on blog
Hang out with encouraging friends

PHYSICAL ACTIVITY
If it rains, indoor activities
  like crunches
Ride bike for thirty minutes
Pant and sweat
Join the basketball team

MOTIVATION
Nonfood rewards—nail polish
Read inspirational autobiographies

By identifying these simple practices and making a plan to implement them at home, the camp attempted to prepare the campers to transfer their camp-acquired habits (and self-control) to their home environments. It is unlikely, however, that these small, detailed changes could overpower the greater influences of the family and cultural practices to which the child would return.

Discussion

The camp wanted the children to attribute weight management to effort and was focused on getting the kids to change their locus of control and regard their body weight as controllable. If effective, their effort to manage weight would be permanent and maintained to the point that the new habits would become ingrained in their personality. The camp was socializing the children not merely to adopt new habits but also to change their personalities. Beliefs and behaviors that aligned with weight management were lauded as being attributes of a certain type of person—specifically, one who can manage his or her weight. By describing concrete methods to change the way they think about themselves and their habits, the children were encouraged to develop a certain kind of self that was internally motivated to change behavior and face challenges with a positive and patient attitude.

The children provided explanations that went beyond the camp's focus on effort and self-control. The campers also attributed weight to family habits, emotional eating and psychological problems, medical problems, and "just luck." Neither the camp nor the children provided structural, cultural, or environmental explanations for weight. All the attributions were at the level of the individual or family. Without taking seriously causes related to the food system, environmental toxins, or social class, the campers were left with a view of weight that was ultimately personal and that left them with the conclusion that their weight was either controllable by them or the result of their bad luck.

6

Change Your Body,
Change Yourself

Camp Resocialization

Steve, the camp director, brought the scale to the cabin porch. One by one, the campers stepped on the scale. The number was covered with an index card so they could not see their weight right away. A counselor recorded it on their chart, and Steve promised to tell them their weight later if they wanted to know. A few hours later, Fay, the other camp director, went to their cabins with a clipboard and the results of the weigh-in. She asked the campers, one at a time, in private, how they felt, and if they had noticed any differences in their energy level, body, and sense of fitness. Then she told them their weight.

The weekly weigh-in was by far the most emotionally charged moment at camp. While Fay attempted to frame the weight loss results as one measure among many, the campers emphasized the number of pounds lost over holistic or subjective measures. After they returned to the porch, they told the others—or not—depending on how much weight they had lost. The campers were always curious to know how many pounds everyone else lost, but some were hesitant to share their own low numbers. A counselor said, "Remember, don't compare yourself to others," and Jasmine replied sarcastically, "Oh, I thought it was a competition." The counselor then told them that numbers don't matter; what matters is that you feel good about yourself. In fact, the numbers did matter to the campers and visibly influenced their emotional expressions. High amounts of weight loss led to feelings of pride and accomplishment, whereas low amounts resulted in frustration and disappointment.

To say that the main objective of a weight loss camp is to have its participants lose weight may seem like an obvious point. There is no doubt that the participants wanted to lose weight, and the camp staff wanted to help them to lose weight. Yet, within the local culture of Camp Odyssey, the meanings of bodily change became far more complex and nuanced as people negotiated the challenging realities of weight loss. The camp emphasized subjective well-being as a benefit of weight loss, although there was a clear tension between objective and subjective measures for both the campers and the camp leaders.

The camp was set up to resocialize the children by teaching them to implement a body project. There were three dimensions to the body project that the camp proposed. First, the traditional dieting model was present. This idea is based on the energy balance model, which supposes that weight can be maintained by consuming and expending an equal amount of calories, and weight loss occurs through a caloric deficit by restricting calories and/or increasing physical activity. Second, the camp also occasionally relied on the Health At Every Size model, which advocates for the pursuit of health and fitness regardless of body weight. Finally, messages related to well-being, character, self-control, and morality were intermingled with the weight loss and fitness objectives. This chapter details how the camp conveyed these messages and socialized the children to adopt them, the responses of the campers to these messages, and the broader implications of socializing children to implement these three aspects of the weight loss camp's body project.

Resocialization as a Body Project

A children's weight loss camp is a setting for resocialization programming. Resocialization is a process of learning a new set of internalized norms, beliefs, and behaviors in order to transform a status or identity created by previous socialization. Research on resocialization often centers on adults who undergo processes of either occupational socialization, such as becoming a doctor or police officer,[1] or institutionalization, such as becoming a prisoner or a mental patient.[2] The focus on adults in resocialization research is so pervasive that it is sometimes referred to as "adult socialization."[3] Most research on childhood focuses on primary socialization processes, that is, how children engage with dominant cultural meanings and learn social order through interaction. While sociologists argue that young people are active and agentic participants in bridging adult and peer cultures through social interaction, the idea of children intentionally attempting to overcome their previous socialization while still in childhood has not been adequately examined.[4]

Resocialization aimed at weight loss can take a number of forms, ranging from dieting on one's own to online or in-person support groups. Erving Goffman's foundational concept of a "total institution," a completely controlled environment with an elaborate system of punishments and rewards aimed at producing conformity and reform, is an ideal type of resocialization that is most useful for thinking about asylums and prisons.[5] A weight loss camp resembles a total institution due to high levels of social control. The daily schedule of activities as well as when and what to eat are strictly regulated by those in power: the camp directors and counselors. Campers are removed from the outside world and permitted limited contact with other influential agents of socialization, such as family, peers, and media. However, there are important differences. In contrast to a total institution like a prison, the children's weight loss camp is a voluntary resocialization program aimed at intense change in a short period of time. While prisoners are held against their will and may resist rehabilitation, a weight loss camp relies on the supposition that its participants are motivated to seek involvement in their own resocialization. Therefore, weight loss camps are best conceptualized as a blend of external social control factors and individual investments in self-change through the implementation of a body project.

Body projects are ongoing processes in which people shape and maintain their body through vigilant effort and techniques, such as diet, exercise, or cosmetic surgery. Body projects require intentional and strategic attempts to change habits and the self. Individual responsibility and self-expression are implicated in body projects as people are "conscious of and actively concerned about the management, maintenance, and appearance of their bodies."[6] Body projects related to weight management are typically based on the dominant energy balance model (i.e., calories in versus calories out), which occurs at the level of individual responsibility and obscures broader social systems that may contribute to increased body size in the population, such as social inequality, the food system, and a neoliberal political system.[7] This focus on individual responsibility for body size persists despite the fact that over 80 percent of U.S. adults fail to maintain weight loss within a year.[8]

At Camp Odyssey, the campers were involved in a carefully packaged regimen of diet, exercise, and educational activities. In doing so, an important aspect of resocialization was explicitly guiding children toward new habits, skills, and knowledge so that they enact bodily and self-change in order to attain weight loss. Campers learned about balancing "regular" and "real" foods as well as visualization strategies related to portion control. The camp provided the background information that would be necessary to change habits into a long-term lifestyle based on day to day food choices.

When "Not a Diet" Is Actually a Diet

The primary way that the camp socialized the children to diet was to restrict portion sizes. During education sessions, campers were taught strategies related to portion control. The visiting dietician provided visualization techniques to teach portion size. She told them that most people fill up their entire plate with spaghetti, but one serving of spaghetti should fit in the palm of your hand. Then she engaged them in active learning by telling them to cup their hand in order to visualize what one serving is. Next, she told everyone to make a fist and place it under their heart. She said, "That is the size of your stomach. It is the size of a pear, but it can expand to go as big as you stuff it."

The MyPlate method, which had recently replaced the food pyramid as the government's nutritional symbol, was another prominent educational tool presented to the campers. The MyPlate method is a visual of a sectioned plate. Half of the plate is fruits and vegetables, a quarter of the plate is protein, and a quarter is grains or carbs, and a side of low-fat dairy is symbolized by a glass of milk. When asked to list what types of foods are proteins, grains, fruits, and vegetables, the campers excelled at coming up with the appropriate responses. However, during the third week, the campers found it difficult to create meal plans using the MyPlate method. While they could easily call out types of foods, they struggled to come up with a day's worth of meals and mostly named meals that they had eaten the day before at camp. While campers were able to gain knowledge, they sometimes had difficulty applying it to real-life situations.

Eating "real foods" was emphasized by basing meals on fresh, nonprocessed food and encouraging campers to try new food through cooking and tasting demonstrations. However, camp leaders did not want the children to feel like they were deprived of food that children would typically eat. Therefore, small amounts of junk food, such as baked chips or popsicles, were provided as a snack. Nicole told them that the way they eat at camp is not a diet because they eat the food that everyone else eats. Campers were told that there is no good or bad food, just food that you should eat more or less often. Fay addressed why they were permitted to eat junk food by asking, "Why are we allowed to have it? You can eat all of this because of the portion. You can have your chips, your ice cream. We just are not overdoing it."

When I asked the campers what they learned at camp, many of them brought up the idea that no food is off limits so long as it is portion controlled. Ryan described the camp by saying "They don't deprive you of anything. You can eat quite a bit of taste good food, you just eat less of it." Ada said, "This camp, it's kind of like a diet, but it's like, how can I say it without making it sound like, it's a diet but it's not depriving you of anything." The campers readily identified the energy balance model that the camp espoused. Faith learned, "You should always read the labels on things and have meals and snacks about 300 calories so you eat less than you are used to. And you're supposed to get 60 minutes of exercise every day."

There were areas of resistance that the campers displayed in reaction to these socialization processes. Despite being told that real food was better for them and that they were not being deprived of junk food, campers talked about food that was not offered to them at camp, such as pizza and peanut butter sandwiches. As their time at camp progressed, these conversations about the food they missed from home increased in frequency. While certainly more reasonable than the grueling boot camp of military-style drills and tasteless food that many of the children imagined as alternative styles to Camp Odyssey, teaching the children to eat small portions of junk food presupposes a great deal of self-control. At camp, the portions were controlled for them, but some campers knew it would be far more difficult to stop eating delicious food when on their own.

A few of the older girls recognized that they would have to be able to eventually make their own food choices and did not feel entirely prepared to do so. On a rare occasion when the campers were not told what to eat at a picnic with Camp Jay, Kelly explained, "When we had lunch on Saturday, and we had to make our own choices, they threw us in there. I totally blanked on what were starches and what was protein. I had no idea what to grab. They were like, this is a test." She also admitted that "at home, I'd probably definitely have seconds or thirds and not just eat the one serving that they give us." Janet said, "I wish there was a way that you could be taught personal pressure like that. . . . this is a big thing, it doesn't improve your personal pressure to be looking at food and resist it if what's actually holding you back from that food is actually social pressure." Here, Janet points out that the camp was not really teaching willpower so much as it was enforcing the children's "choices" through social control.

Further, the juxtaposition of healthy and junk food reflects broader tensions within dieting culture when the social value of a thin body competes with the contemporary food environment. Susan Bordo refers to the broad psychopathologies of food and diet that have caused a widespread "cultural bulimia" in which people are told to indulge in decadent, calorie-dense foods and also to maintain a slender physique through diet and exercise.[9] Thus both epidemic anorexia and obesity "are rooted in the same consumer-culture construction of desire as overwhelming and overtaking the self. Given that construction, we can only respond either with total submission or rigid defense."[10] While the camp attempted to find a middle ground, it may have unwittingly reinforced notions of willpower in the face of junk food temptation which were unrealistic outside the controlled environment of camp.

Embodied Resocialization

In addition to providing strategies and knowledge to influence decision making, weight loss resocialization also involves embodiment, the physical sensations that come to feel natural through socialization. Resocialization must also focus on the mind–body connection so that changes become a physically rooted, normal way of being for the person. For example, Loic Wacquant's research as a participant observer at a boxing gym on Chicago's South Side demonstrates how boxers experience embodied change via an environment supportive of specific training techniques as well as careful practices and strategies.[11] Through various kinds of labor, such as physical training to punch efficiently, emotion work to control fear and anger in the ring, and using time and rhythm to allow the body to pace itself during a three-minute round, individuals condition their bodies to behave as boxers. When this training is successful, the mind and body are integrated to the point that a boxer can go on fighting even if he is semiconscious.

Like Wacquant's boxers, the dieting and fitness regimen at a weight loss camp may entail conscious choices and learning but will be deemed successful self-change only when the child manages cravings and reduces the amount of food eaten in a way that comes to feel natural and normal. Body size and weight loss concerns speak directly to the issue of embodiment—merging cognition and sensation, thoughts, and a sense of well-being as people attempt to simultaneously change their thought patterns and physical reactions.

The camp staff recognized that changing eating habits is not solely based on learning facts about nutrition and portion control. Therefore, campers were taught to make the connection between their thoughts and embodiment by recalibrating hunger and practicing mindful eating. The first lesson at camp dealt with the hunger scale. The hunger scale ranged from 1 to 10, with 1 being ravenously hungry and 10 being painfully stuffed. They were told that they should always maintain their hunger levels between 3 (hungry) and 6 (full) with 5 being pleasantly satisfied. Fay regularly asked if anyone had been feeling hungry or how full they were at that moment. Most said they were 4 or 5. Sometimes, they provided specific numbers, such as 4.7 or 5.3. During the entire time at camp, I never heard campers say they were a number outside the acceptable 4 to 6 range.

Fay explained that the purpose of the hunger scale was to allow campers to check in with their body and to maintain self-control over how much they ate. The link between the mind and the body was made explicit when Fay said, "You need to change your thinking so that a 5 feels good." Using the hunger scale as a cognitive tool and labeling a certain level of satiety as "good," the body will feel different, and overeating will be unappealing, if not intolerable. Fay told them that if she or one of the counselors overeats, they feel so uncomfortable that they cannot stand it, and they do not want to do that again. By not overeating, campers were told that they would experience other embodied benefits, such as being able to move, feeling energetic, and feeling good about themselves. Fay told them that if they could sell themselves on feeling comfortable at a 5, they would be more successful when they returned home.

The hunger scale was a popular tool among the campers who used it even without staff prompting. However, the program leaders had to adjust their teaching to clarify that saying you are not hungry was only a good thing if you were eating adequately. There was an acceptable yet amorphous amount of hunger and food that campers were permitted. While most campers did not ask for more food, a few were reprimanded for not eating enough. For example, Jenny did not finish all her food at breakfast one morning. Fay saw this and said, "Jenny, you hardly ate anything." Jenny replied, "I'm not hungry." Fay said in a disapproving tone, "You haven't been eating very much." After Fay walked away, Jenny turned to her friends and said, "Fay got mad at me for not eating." Here, we see an example of the confusion that campers had when they followed the guidelines to eat less, and the concern among adults that some were not eating enough. During the last week of camp, the issue of the girls not eating enough was addressed at their Education session. The counselors told the girls that their level of activity required them to take in enough calories for energy, and the camp provided a good amount of food, not too much or too little, but they had to eat what was provided.

In addition to teaching campers what to eat, the camp staff also tried to retrain *how* campers ate. They adopted an approach called Mindful Eating. A counselor explained that Mindful Eating focuses on hunger and fullness cues; centers attention on the mental, physical, and emotional effects of food; and instills a positive regard for food. The Mindful Eating style is in contrast to the assumed mindless overeating style that the campers had acquired before camp. Mindful Eating connects mental awareness and embodied habits, such as taste, chewing, and eating slowly. Campers experienced Mindful Eating through a taste test. They were given fruit, a cracker, and a piece of chocolate and told to look at and smell each one. Then they were guided to eat each piece of food mindfully—first putting it in their mouth and letting it sit there, then chewing it slowly before swallowing it. The children responded enthusiastically to this exercise and commented that food tasted differently when they slowed down. A few of the boys contrasted this experience to the past when they put handfuls of crackers or chocolates in their mouth at one time. By adding an embodied experience to verbal instruction about Mindful Eating, the program facilitated a connection between the mind and the body.

Chewing slowly was a consistent message during the Education sessions and at meals. The counselors often led the campers to sing about chewing before meals. The lyrics were set to the tune of "Row, Row, Row Your Boat":

Chew, chew, chew your food
Slowly through your meal
The more you chew, the less you eat
The better you will feel.

At the end of the first week, Fay issued a challenge for the day. She told the campers to take a bite and count how many chews they normally took before swallowing. Then, for the next bite, they should add ten chews. The next day when she asked them how they did with the challenge, she was met with resistance. One camper said that by chewing so much, the food disappears or tastes gross when it liquefies. Fay amended her advice and told them to add only a few extra chews from now on.

The camp thus attempted to retrain the campers' sense of the mind–body connection so that they would eat less food and change their style of eating. Just as Wacquant's boxers trained to fight in strategic and purposeful ways that eventually became habitual and embodied, the campers learned that weight loss also requires a reciprocal mind–body connection. The program explained how weight management operates through physiological cues, such as hunger and fullness. The campers were then taught to use mental strategies to become aware of their body's cues. The program assumed that the children had been overeating because they were overriding their body's signals of fullness. Through the recalibration of hunger that occurred during their time at camp, the intent was that the body would feel better and send new signals to the brain. Specifically, both the mind and the body would be more satisfied with less food and healthier types of food. The program introduced a new target of satiety, gave the body time to adjust, and trained the campers to view this new level of fullness as desirable. While the campers participated in and largely enjoyed the taste tests, the songs, and the hunger scale, these tactics still required their active negotiation as participants constructed new meanings related to hunger and navigated behaviors such as chewing slowly.

Substituting Outcomes: Fitness or Thinness?

Another dimension of the body project that the camp attempted to instill in the children was the idea that physical fitness was an important outcome. The focus on health and fitness provided an alternative to weight loss through food restriction, and it served as an important coping strategy when confronted with the flaws of dieting. The high failure rate causes some people to reject the

premise of dieting to lose weight altogether. The Health At Every Size philosophy posits that people should focus on nutrition and exercise instead of
attaining weight loss in order to fit medicalized BMI categories.[12] Additionally, physical activity, whether one is pursuing weight reduction or size
acceptance, denotes morality even if one does not attain the cultural body size
ideal. The meaning of body size at a weight loss camp—where the objective to
attain a thin body may seem straightforward—required sophisticated
negotiation and hedging techniques by both the program and its participants.

Each day, the campers went swimming and had the opportunity to participate in a variety of exercises that changed daily, such as kickboxing or
yoga. The camp was so large that the campers also walked long distances to go
between activities, the cafeteria, and the cabins. At the end of the first week,
the staff informed the campers that they were walking 5K every day just getting
from place to place. In this way, the campers were becoming fit without realizing
it because walking around camp was not officially labeled movement. Fay often
used the phrase "hooked on fitness," meaning that people who are active cannot
go a day without moving because it becomes normal. She wanted them to get
addicted to movement and the feeling of activity. When they were forced to
live in an active way, their bodies adapted. Once again, the importance of
embodied change for resocialization is highlighted. Fay recognized that
willpower is just a small part, but noticing changes in their body and experiencing new feelings of wellness could be the incentive to make permanent behavioral changes.

While acknowledging the importance of weight loss, the program directors
introduced fitness as a simultaneous outcome. Unquestionably, the camp
directors wanted the campers to attain *both* weight loss and fitness. However,
in terms of attainability and morale, the benefits of emphasizing fitness proved
important. From the beginning of camp, the directors hedged when it came to
saying that weight loss and becoming thin were the ultimate goals. They told
the campers' parents that they believed people can be healthy at any weight,
and they wanted to deemphasize weight. Instead, they encouraged the campers
to measure success in terms of how they felt, their energy levels, and fitness. The
children completed a fitness pretest and posttest consisting of push-ups, sit-ups,
and a 1-mile walk/run.

While fitness and weight loss can go hand in hand, the message about their
relative importance and relationship was confusing at times. For example, a day
before the first week's weigh-in, Fay said they should not emphasize how much
weight they lost, but rather how much their fitness had improved. She asked
them how many pounds they thought people would lose. The campers guessed
between 1 and 6 pounds. Then she said, "Don't compare yourself to what others
have lost, just focus on fitness. You can be fit and heavy. However, that doesn't
mean it's okay to be heavy. You can still get diseases—not that you have diseases

now but you can be at risk for them, and it can become that way if you are overweight. But it is better if you are heavy and fit."

In this exchange, Fay told them not to focus on numbers but then immediately asked them to guess a number for pounds lost. Then she responded to those numbers by saying that being overweight is unhealthy, yet fitness is more important than weight loss. Thus they should focus on fitness more than weight—but they should still try to lose weight. Fay encouraged them to focus on fitness as a dimension of health even if they were overweight. Here, we see an implicit bodily hierarchy emerge. Being thin and fit was at the top, and this was what the program believed should be their aspiration. However, the reality was that achieving thinness may be a long process and one that cannot be guaranteed. Therefore, the next best alternative was to be overweight and physically fit. The implication was that being overweight and unfit was unacceptable, so the campers had to meet one of these objectives as part of their body project at camp.

Objective measures of weight loss were important to the staff and meaningful to the campers. Yet, even when a camper was successful with weight loss, Fay connected it to fitness. When Jenny said that she walks faster and sweats more, Fay responded that those were nice changes because they were related to movement and not just about clothes fitting. While many of the campers were excited about aesthetic and weight changes, Fay often tried to shift their focus to fitness. Invoking fitness and well-being points to the benefits of pursuing weight loss regardless of whether people actually lose weight. By framing the process in a positive way as being physically rewarding and focusing on physical changes other than weight loss, the camp provided subjective meanings of implementing a body project that could be immediately deployed to raise spirits.

Health Concerns, Healthism, and Scare Tactics

The construction of the healthy body involves a self-care regimen aimed at not only preventing disease but also making people feel good about their appearance.[13] The increased attention to health in modern society has been critiqued by scholars who argue that it creates a discriminatory system they refer to as "healthism."[14] Healthism posits that the pursuit of health has become a moral imperative, a marker of being a good person, and a matter of individual responsibility. The campers brought health concerns with them to camp, but the camp also fostered alarm regarding medical conditions that they associated with weight, especially diabetes.

Bridget said she wanted to lose weight "to be healthier and live longer." Sarah said that she did not want health problems or diabetes. Some saw the health problems faced by family members as a cautionary tale. Tom said, "On my dad's side, diabetes runs in the family real bad. One day my grandpa couldn't feel his foot. They found out his sugar level was so low." Mandy worried about her health. She said, "I kind of think, what is going to happen if I keep gaining pounds? Is my metabolism just going to shut down? Am I going to have to take a lot of pills? That's what my grandma and my great grandma have, and my mom has it. My mom said she never exercised when it happened, so if I keep going, it'll keep going and won't shut down."

Several campers told me that their doctors told them to lose weight, and they had already faced health problems. Zach's weight impacted his health. He explained, "Last year, I had an appendix thing, but it was a false alarm. I went to the hospital, and the doctor was talking about surgery. And it would be kind of hard, though, because of my weight. So they put me on an 1800-calorie diet, which was really hard." Ray had a series of health problems that caused him to be hospitalized, including a hip infection. He explained, "I have something called a shunt inside of me where it drains brain fluid down to here. I can't play football. There are certain sports I can't play like soccer. It really pains me because I know I could easily play the sports. It is directly affected by my weight. Overweight people are more prone to the disease."

Jasmine was diagnosed with diabetes when she was 9 years old and had been hospitalized frequently due to diabetic complications and sleep apnea.

My doctor and aunt told me if I don't lose weight, I might lose an arm or something like that because of my diabetes. When I was in the hospital, I was afraid to eat at all. I didn't want to move around because the pain would go to my leg and make my leg hurt and everything was sitting on my nervous system. . . . I was at the hospital a lot though. In and out. In and out. Before I knew I had diabetes, I had sleep apnea. I had to get surgery. I had to get my tonsils and adenoids out. . . . I want to be off my diabetes forever. I'm tired of poking myself in the stomach and the fingers every day. I'm tired of going to the doctor almost every week.

Several other campers reported that their doctors either warned them of diabetes due to their weight or had diagnosed them as prediabetic. While only a handful of campers had weight-related health issues, their experiences and fear of negative health repercussions loomed large at camp.

At camp, Jasmine's blood sugar was hard to manage, and she said it was even harder to control at home. During the first week, there was a staff meeting about Jasmine's diabetes. Her blood sugar reading that morning was over 400. They consulted with a nurse practitioner who explained to them the dangers of diabetes and the consequences of high blood sugar. Jasmine had eaten French toast and fruit for breakfast, so they assessed that there might be too much sugar in the camp diet for a diabetic.

While there was some discussion of avoiding foods that are high in fat, such as when Sam went over "dangers of the salad bar" like high-fat dressings and toppings, the chief nutritional bogeyman of camp was sugar. There was a high level of interest for two reasons. First, the emphasis on real foods allowed for healthy fats, and they mentioned several times that the low-fat diet movement only caused people to gain weight because of added sugars. Second, Fay was in charge of managing Jasmine's diabetes and became particularly interested in learning more about it and educating the campers. This culminated in a physician coming in as a guest speaker to teach the campers about diabetes.

Dr. Redd asked the campers to participate in a demonstration using a water park as an analogy. She told them to pretend that they were outside a water park waiting to enter. Jenny volunteered to be the ticket taker. Dr. Redd instructed five campers to be well behaved as they walked through the ticket gate where Jenny handed them tickets. Dr. Redd pointed out that the orderliness allowed them to get in without Jenny working too hard. She told the next group of five campers to be rowdy because they had no parents with them. She asked Jenny if she would be able to keep up if kids like that were coming in all day. Jenny said no. Finally, she had five rowdy campers go through the line after being paired with a counselor. She said that there were more people, but it was orderly again.

After the campers returned to their seats, Dr. Redd explained the analogy. The ticket taker is the pancreas, the kids are sugar, the ticket is insulin, and the waterpark is the cell. When there is too much sugar, the extra sugar molecules do not get absorbed, and they sit in the bloodstream. High blood sugar means that the sugar is attached to the walls and is not circulating. Fat and cholesterol come to clean it up, and this narrows blood vessels, causing damage to the heart, kidneys, and feet because nerves die. She said that you should worry about diabetes because of the vessel damage that can lead to kidney failure, dialysis, loss of sight, and amputation. Jasmine, the diabetic camper, listed a lot of these consequences, and the doctor said, "You're the expert."

Dr. Redd said that diabetes cannot be reversed, but it can be slowed down. It may take ten years for a blockage to form when someone has full-blown diabetes. She said that insulin resistance can be reversed, but you have to lower the amount of sugar you eat so that your pancreas can catch up. She then explained that people should eat carbohydrates along with protein and fiber to act as chaperones. This point was further elaborated at the next education session by the dietician who gave examples of partnering proteins, such as eating eggs and toast instead of a pop-tart for breakfast. The next day, Fay reviewed the doctor's analogy. She said that when people eat too many carbohydrates, the body turns it into fat for storage and the "real reason you end up overweight is that your body can't handle it." Then she asked the campers to name one thing they learned at camp, and it was clear that the recentness and urgency of the message affected some of their answers. For example, Gabe said, "Sugar overloads the pancreas" and Charlie said, "Do not overload on sugar or you will get diabetes." Fay responded, "That is really the problem."

I attended and took notes at every Education session during camp. The vast majority of the time, I found that the nutritional guidance was fairly straightforward. The staff, at times, even made an additional effort to lessen shame or negative talk regarding food and eating (such as telling the children that there are not "good" or "bad" foods). My main critique was that some of their weight loss rhetoric was contradictory or disingenuous in that they claimed that it was a lifestyle change when it really was a controlled diet. However, the diabetes lectures by the guest speakers and then the way Fay referred to sugar and diabetes in the following days disturbed me. I wrote in my field notes, "The Education session today was a scary and very shaming medical talk about diabetes. I felt bad for Jasmine." I have no doubt that Fay was curious and concerned about diabetes for Jasmine's sake, yet the delivery of the information was insensitive and over the top. Diabetes was constructed as a frightening medical condition that would sabotage life and limbs without concern for Jasmine's feelings, given that all of the campers were aware that she had diabetes. Further, it genuinely scared the campers as it linked their body weight to diabetes and imposed the imperative of weight loss for health. I interviewed Melissa a few hours after the diabetes lecture, and she was clearly shaken from the information presented.

MELISSA: I don't want to get a disease or a stroke or a heart attack or diabetes.
LB: Did that talk really affect you this morning?
MELISSA: Yeah, I'm so scared now. I don't want to be like that.

The camp used scare tactics to link health and weight. For the campers who faced genuine health issues, the camp's discussion of their health challenges was shaming rather than helpful. By equating the unhealthy body with fear and shame, the camp reinforced the notion that children's bodies were problems that needed to be solved.

Body Projects and Being a Certain Kind of Person

Linking body weight to self-control and morality is culturally deep seated. Obesity is especially likely to be framed as a morality tale focusing on personal responsibility and blame in the United States.[15] While the social value of thinness may be an incentive for people to engage in weight control tactics, the high failure rate of dieting points to the idea that body projects provide ancillary functions beyond successful bodily change. In addition to encouraging behavioral and attitudinal change, weight loss programs provide valuable emotional support and social services as well as organized frames for people to deal with weight-related shame, either through avowal or contestation.[16] Further, the pursuit of weight loss aligns with the values espoused by healthism in which putting forth effort to change one's body reflects worth, self-control, and deservingness. Thus dieting and physical activity can be used to signal a person's character regardless of his or her body size. The camp's body project centered on self-improvement. The implementation of a body project was linked to being the type of person who values personal responsibility. Beliefs and behaviors that were aligned with the objectives of thinness and fitness became their own measure of success, even if bodily transformation did not occur. Character and self-change served as another possible way to implement a body project.

Self-control was regarded as an important part of the body project. Fay said, "I'm serious when kids go home and haven't practiced this muscle—they haven't learned to push the food away or move. You have to work on self-control." The children were taught that control over one's body was the way to achieve high self-esteem and attain thinness and fitness. The corollary was that being overweight was a character flaw indicative of a passive, lazy, and out of control person. By placing weight management solely at the level of individual responsibility and conflating self-control with body size, the camp reinforced messages that ultimately stigmatize heavy people.

Despite the camp's use of objective measures, like weekly weigh-ins, Fay frequently asked the children to focus on subjective feelings, which are internally defined and cannot be measured by others, such as energy levels and feeling "good." When Jasmine gained a pound one week, the response was an attempt to salvage positive meaning and to show that she was still making progress in self-change. Jasmine said that she did not feel like she got much accomplished because of the weight gain. Fay asked the other girls if they had noticed changes in Jasmine's body. The other girls piped up that she was doing a lot more physically and trying hard. Fay agreed that gaining a pound can be discouraging, but she recommended that Jasmine focus on the other benefits she was getting from camp and to be proud of her effort.

Although rare, the failure to attain weight loss was a tricky moment of emotion management at camp. Campers who did not lose weight were upset that the program was not working at that point. Offering words of encouragement and comfort, they praised qualities such as effort even if the body did not respond to their desires and attempts to change it. The program and its participants had to salvage meaning by shifting the focus from outcomes to how valiant the attempt to change was. Attention was diverted to acknowledging hard work and effort, and promoting alternative definitions of success based on character and self-change. Had the adults not been able to maintain a positive morale by providing plausible alternatives to weight loss, the children may have resisted the program directives.

Resocialization through Social Control

Camp Odyssey believed that its effectiveness was largely rooted in the immersive environment that allowed children to "recalibrate" their past habits. Self-control not only occurred through intentionally changing thought patterns, it was also *experienced* through being part of a new environment. The immersive environment greatly contributed to the camp's resocialization program. The camp philosophy was that resetting hunger, activity level, and tastes would be easier without the temptations, distractions, and established routines of home. The hope was that when they returned home, their time at camp would have fundamentally reset who they were so that they would react differently to their former environment. This implies a view that self-control, once established, will transfer to other environments.

While the immersive environment of camp afforded recalibration of past habits, this also created reliance on social control mechanisms. The camp carefully controlled food options and portion sizes. Before every meal, the group formed a circle outside of the cafeteria to listen to announcements and sing the chewing song. Then a counselor brought over a sample plate to show what foods they could eat and the appropriate portion sizes. During meals, counselors policed the salad bar and the entrée at the table. If a camper took too many beans or not enough vegetables, they would be verbally reprimanded. Staff particularly monitored how much salad dressing the campers poured. While the campers could serve themselves, they were not allowed to choose how much they served. Some complained, but they also became reliant on this guidance. In addition to this direct form of social control, there was enormous social pressure not to ask for more food. Rarely, a child asked a counselor for permission to get more food or another piece of fruit. If it was not a vegetable request (which was always accepted), they were often told no.

During free time, the counselors checked in with the campers about their eating and exercise habits. One counselor, Sam, had a reputation for interrogating the campers about their past habits at home and what they were doing at camp. While some of the campers were annoyed by his style, others recognized his function. When writing goals for home, a few girls talked about making a cutout of Sam to watch over them while they eat at home. One suggested that they create a "Sam-bot" that would robotically tell them what they should be eating and doing, and it would make them feel guilty if they made the wrong choices. This exchange shows that the girls did not fully trust themselves to make food choices at home, and their behavior at camp was largely driven by staff surveillance rather than self-directed decision making.

Since campers did not choose what they were eating, the camp had complete control over providing only foods that fit with their nutritional model. Eating what was provided allowed the campers' tastes to be recalibrated by the camp environment, but it also meant that they did not make food-related decisions about cutting calories and restricting portions like they would if dieting at home. Within this environmental control, the children lost weight. However, the long-term prospects for self-change were limited because their success was a product of the structured environment. While the children were able to change their habits at camp, these changes were linked to camp surveillance. When faced with a noncamp environment, their new habits were put to the test.

Testing the Resocialization Process

Reentry into the noncamp world was fraught with challenges. The contrast between controlled camp life to noncamp "real" life was experienced for the first time when the campers spent the day at a water park at the end of the second week. The water park revealed how the camp-sanctioned narrative of embodied change was parroted by campers and yet was ultimately ineffective when the campers were faced with making eating decisions on their own.

Fay predicted that the campers' choices at the water park would show how much they had changed, and she acknowledged that the campers often said the right things without actually believing or practicing it. The water park was an opportunity to test the effectiveness of the camp's resocialization efforts. The day before the water park, Fay told the campers they would have five dollars to spend, and there would be cheese fries, ice cream, chili dogs, and onion rings at the water park. She said to think about whether they feel pressured to eat because it is available and to keep in mind "that's the way the world is. We want you to have five dollars so that you have practice in the real world."

Fay reminded the campers to think about the hunger/fullness scale when they made their decision. She repeated that it was up to them to practice decision making, and if they were full, they could throw the food away. Then Fay revisited the camp-sanctioned narrative about their changed habits and selves. She said that in past years kids came back to camp feeling ill due to eating junk food. Throughout camp, the kids were told that their tastes were changing, and they would find junk food much sweeter or greasier after they became used to healthy eating. Fay invoked campers' agency in decision making and managing portions by throwing away food if they were full. She drew on resocialization strategies like the hunger scale and the embodied consequences of eating junk food. The camp narrative was meant to show the children that their tastes had been reset to the point that they would find their old eating habits and food choices unappealing.

When they returned from the water park, Fay met with the campers to discuss how they had handled food at the water park. She said she wanted them to have this experience so they could gain awareness about themselves because "being at home is like being at a water park every day." Some of the campers drew on the camp narrative that had been previously discussed. For example, Sarah said that she split cheese fries with three other people. Even though it was a small portion, she felt sick because of the salt and fat, and it was "just gross. I'm done with fries. My mouth felt greasy." Ada said that the French fries did not taste like she thought they would. Fay replied, "I'm not surprised because taste buds change." Ada said she soon found herself hungry again and this was a "terrible feeling." From the camp program's perspective, campers who expressed both mental and physical aversion to unhealthy food had successfully achieved resocialization.

For others, confronting food choices at the water park was a challenge. Kelly reported feeling "weird" when she decided on ice cream and asked herself, "Should I be eating something else? Nothing?" When confronted with the food options, Sasha recalled telling herself, "No, you can't have this. You have to eat healthy. This is bad for you." In direct violation of the camp narrative, a couple girls ate junk food despite not liking it. Kyra bought mini corn dogs that she did not like, but she ate them anyway. Jasmine ordered cheese fries and admitted that even though she didn't like the way they tasted, "I kept putting it in my mouth. The taste got stuck, and I couldn't stop."

Despite being provided a packed, Odyssey-approved lunch, every single camper ate some type of food at the park. Most of them used negative words like "gross" or "disgusting" to describe it. When campers expressed a neutral or positive reaction to the junk food, Fay disapproved because she wanted them to embrace the narrative that their tastes had changed, and they did not like that type of food anymore. The majority of the campers used the camp-approved narrative indicating they now preferred healthy food and the camp lifestyle. However, not all campers said those things, and even those who did still ate junk food. The camp narrative was not completely preventive, especially for campers who continued to eat junk food that did not taste good.

Visitors Day

Although Fay likened the water park to the "real" world, the amusement park confections did not reflect their typical home environment. One of the most revealing tests that the campers faced was when parents visited and took the campers away for the day. Most of the families went to a restaurant for a big meal. A few went to a nearby sit-down restaurant known for its elk burgers. One went to a Chinese buffet. Many campers reported that their family members ordered appetizers. Kyra did not eat any of the appetizers her mother ordered because she remembered how full she was at the water park and did not want to repeat that experience. Others could not resist. When her family ordered artichoke spinach dip, Ada told them that appetizers make you full before you get your food. After it arrived, though, it looked so good that she tried it with carrots and celery, but then she ate it with the chips. She felt so full that she ate less than half of her entrée. Fay said that it can be a slippery slope when dining out, and she asked Ada if she thought her parents were tempting her. Ada shook her head no and then said "Uh huh, maybe." Fay told her that type of sabotage happens to a lot of campers.

The campers noticed that their families ate a lot faster than they did. Ada said that her mom "pounded a BLT," and Sharon said her mom kept taking fries mindlessly. The practice of eating slowly at camp had taken hold for most of them. Mandy's family took her to Denny's where her brother ordered a burger, fries, and a sundae. Her family had to wait an extra twenty minutes for her to finish eating. Several of the campers noted that they pushed their plate away when they felt full as a strategy. Kelly's father intervened to keep her from snacking on the caramel corn they bought while shopping. She ate some, but it made her feel sick. Her dad held the bag on his other side so she could not reach it. She wanted to have more, but he said, "No, you said you didn't want it." A couple of the campers said they felt sick after drinking soda for the first time in two weeks. Fay told them that taste buds change in two weeks, and you also "feel it in your gut." Janet got a stomach ache and a headache from the soda even though she thought it tasted good. Fay asked her, "Will you be able to hold on to that memory?"

While the campers were able to pinpoint and implement certain strategies they learned at camp, such as eating slowly and pushing food away, they were still placed in highly tempting situations by their families who did not know or practice the strategic elements their children learned during their resocialization at camp. When unhealthy food was in front of them outside the controlled environment of camp, many discovered their impulse was to violate the new eating habits of camp.

Discussion

Weight loss resocialization involves complex processes of conscious intent and direct learning as well as environmental recalibration to form new habits. Camp Odyssey engaged children in a body project and taught them new skills, knowledge, and habits related to nutrition, portion size, and physical activity. The program also provided an environment for children to reset the connection between their mind and body. Techniques aimed at getting children to recalibrate their hunger and use a different style of eating moved beyond the realm of intentional and strategic action to include embodied change.

Childhood is a rich time for taking on cultural meanings, so the camp's strategies related to implementing a body project were readily accepted. It is likely that children are particularly receptive to adding new skills, habits, and strategies to make sense of their lives and to solve problems. Other than a few examples of resistance in the process (e.g., complaining that chewing too much made food "gross"), the campers were sincere in their desire to follow the camp staff's directives in order to lose weight. They wanted to believe in the camp's messages and effectiveness. Along the same lines, children may already be primed to accept adult power and influence over their lives, which makes them more open to resocialization.

In addition to describing these resocialization processes, social control mechanisms and an immersive environment at camp supported resocialization and weight loss in the short term. Indeed, all campers lost weight. However, the long-term effectiveness of the camp's resocialization efforts is unlikely as evidenced by their brief encounters with the outside world during camp. When the children left camp for a water park excursion, it was clear that many could identify features of resocialization in a camp-sanctioned narrative, but they found it difficult to enact these changes without the support and control of the camp. As the camp staff acknowledged, camp was not a "magic bullet." In order for weight loss to be maintained or continued, the resocialization process would have to be adopted by the home environment. The children may have acquired knowledge, achieved physical changes, and experienced a new way of being, but this would not be sustained without adults who continued the camp's resocialization techniques at home.

The most concerning aspect of resocialization at the weight loss camp was that, rather than instilling healthy habits, the experience may have unintentionally set the children up to become lifelong cyclical dieters. While removing the children from their home environments and past habits was effective as a short-term solution, the children were likely to regain the weight upon their return home. This inadvertent yo-yo model of weight management is an unhealthy precedent to set. Research suggests that losing and gaining weight may cause more health problems than being overweight.[17] Further, moralistic undertones and contradictory messages about weight management are unfair to all dieters, but these are particularly burdensome for children. The camp continually told children to work on self-control when, in fact, their weight loss was due in large part to the social control of the camp environment. By teaching children to equate health with morality and sacrifice with self-esteem, the camp sent the message to children that the pursuit of dieting was a valuable—and value-laden—personality trait. In the next chapter, I explore these issues further as I examine the benefits of camp for the children's self-esteem as well as the potentially negative consequences of participating in a weight loss program.

7

The Benefits of Weight Loss Camp . . . and the Dark Side

I'm just so happy that I went to this camp. I can do a lot of things. I'm very athletic. I have a lot of confidence now. In school, I just don't talk to anyone because they are so rude. I love all the activities we do. It's fun. I wish I could stay here forever. With my family.
—Melissa

I'm obviously fat, so it's like, there's no way of telling me that I'm not because I went to a [weight loss] camp. I'm overweight. I need to lose weight. It's just like I couldn't do it any other way. So I think that [bulimia] did the trick a little bit.
—Sharon

How did the camp's messages about weight loss impact the participants' body image and self-esteem? Was the camp a place of fat shaming and disordered eating or did the camp provide a community of belonging that enhanced the children's self-image? Some campers, like Melissa, were wholly positive about their camp experience. Others, like Sharon, were ambivalent about the camp's messages regarding body image and self-change. In this chapter, I explain what the campers viewed as the benefits of attending a weight loss camp. I analyze the campers' body image and the camp's messages about bodily acceptance and change. Then, I examine the underlying "healthism" message at camp and how that impacted the children's self-image. Finally, I contrast Dana and Sharon, the two junior counselors whose self-image differed based on their interpretations and experiences over several years of attending the camp.

The Benefits of Camp

With the exception of Kevin, who dealt with bouts of homesickness, the children were overwhelmingly enthusiastic about their camp experience. When I asked them what they liked about camp, many of the children told me that it was "fun." Specifically, they liked swimming, the activities, and spending time with other campers. Quite a few also told me that they enjoyed learning about nutrition and participating in physical activities.

The camp directors and counselors expressed their intention to create a fun and happy environment for the children, and they seemed to genuinely care about their well-being. As Fay told me in regard to the camp's philosophy, she viewed camp as an opportunity for "kids to be kids" on an even playing field. For Bridget, who at age 11 looked much older due to her height and weight, camp was indeed a place where she was expected to be a kid and not to act like a teenager. She said, "I'm treated like a 13- or 14-year-old when I'm back home, and I'm treated my age here." This was especially powerful given the way that weight could exclude children from typical childhood experiences. Ada was dismayed and embarrassed when her body weight caused her age to be misread at a water park when she was younger: "It was a small slide, so I was like, 'Why can't I go on it?' [The employee said:] 'It's for children. You're like 13.' And I said, 'I'm 9.' It felt really bad. I'm only 9. You just called me a 13-year-old. I feel really bad. I can't go on the slide because I was 1 pound greater than the limit. Now what's up with that? They had scales right there, and they were just looking at us." Whereas the outside world called into question whether she was a child or a teenager due to her weight, Ada saw camp as an encouraging, friendly environment where her body was not hypervisible like it was at the water park slide.

Campers often relayed to me that being around other people who were trying to lose weight was the best part of camp. Ray preferred camp to school because "I think it is a bit more positive because no one is ripping me about my size at least." Zach contrasted his friends at school with his friends at camp. At home, he said, "My friends are not the greatest. If you want to tell something personal, and you're down, no one cares much. They are kind of selfish. Most of my friends are immature." By contrast, at camp, "everyone came here for the same reason, so it is different. You get to know people a lot more because you are with them 24/7 so [you become] closer friends. . . . I guess you tell them personal stuff because they don't really know you. They can't tell your friends at school or anything." Camp made Dana realize that there were better people beyond what she experienced at school. She said, "Last year, I came here, and I had these friends [at school] that I didn't like very well. There are people who are better than that. I met them at camp. I acted how I wanted to at camp, and no one insulted me." Away from the peer cultures and social hierarchies of their schools, the campers felt more accepted.

Another benefit of camp was that it allowed many of the young campers to form a temporary, situational identity. Being away from their families and peers gave them freedom from any prejudgments about who they were. Especially for young people who felt that they did not fit in at school, camp provided a safe haven to speak up more. Sarah explained, "At school, I'm more quiet. . . . At camp, you get to be who you want to be. You try out different personalities." Ada agreed, "At camp, I'm a little more outgoing because I don't really know anybody here. At school, we all knew each other since kindergarten so it's like you can't change personalities." Comparing her behavior at camp to home, Kelly said, "I think I'm a lot more myself. I watch what I say at home, but I think I'm a lot more open here. I share things with people here that I haven't told people at home. I'm a lot more myself. I'm a lot more confident, and I speak up for myself a lot." Dana also said that she acted differently at camp, "At school, I'm a lot more reserved. I don't really talk much at all." As a consequence of problematizing their bodies, many campers suppressed their personalities and became quiet, self-conscious, and closed off. At camp, due to its short-term nature and being around new people who had similar body concerns, the campers felt free to fully express themselves and to be a different version of themselves in a comparatively low-stakes environment.

The camp also provided a way for the young campers to experiment with flirting and romantic relationships. Due to the relatively young average age of the group, there were no serious romances or public displays of affection like there had been in past years. At the end of the first week, Steve mentioned that they usually had to break up camp romances by now. The returning counselors told me that in past years campers snuck into the woods during the mile jog to make out, and they had confiscated sexually explicit letters. Dana, who had attended Camp Odyssey five times, told me that during her first two years, a pair of campers had an ongoing camp relationship that became a prominent matter of discussion among other campers. She said, "There were a lot more relationships then than there are now. Even two years ago, there were a couple of relationships, and last year, there was one or two. This year there aren't that many." Dana described those camp relationships as fairly "juvenile" since they were based on holding hands in public and telling other people that they were dating.

While Ray flirted with Sarah, and there was burgeoning interest between Tom and Kelly over the course of the month, the central romantic drama during camp centered on Sasha. On the way to breakfast on the fourth day of camp, I overheard Sasha and Dustin having a conversation about drinking water instead of soda and writing letters to their families. They sat with each other at the picnic grove before breakfast and walked to activities together that morning. After lunch, Sasha told me that both Ryan and Dustin asked her to the dance, and they had fought to hold the door open for her. Expressing her disbelief that two boys were interested in her, she said, "Is this a dream? I can't believe this is happening." This was especially exciting for her because she had a hard time at school and was often teased by the boys there.

Sasha told everyone that she had been asked to the dance, and her love triangle garnered the attention of the older girls who gossiped about her. It also made the first dance an important subject of speculation. Faith, at only 9 years old, was uncertain about the dance and asked me if you had to have a date and if there were slow dances. I told her that she did not need a date and that it can be fun to go to dances with your friends. The younger girls tried to convince each other to ask the boys to the dance. Jenny and Ada told me about the "Mandy situation," which involved Mandy's crush on Jacob. By the end of the first week, the campers transitioned from same-gender to mixed groups, although contact was still limited and communication between interested parties mostly happened through friends speaking on behalf of others. A simple, short conversation signaled strong interest because they rarely interacted otherwise.

The competition for Sasha's affection led to conflict between Dustin and Ryan. Ryan and Sasha were talking at one end of the pool while Dustin played basketball at the other end. When they were called together to do a group activity, Dustin told Ryan to "stay away from my girl." Ryan replied that she was having second thoughts about him. They proceeded to negotiate that Sasha would go to the dance with Dustin during the first two weeks of camp since he would be leaving, and then she would go with Ryan during the last two weeks since he would be at camp for a month. As this discussion was going on, Jacob was within earshot and moved away, saying "I'm out of here. You are girls now." Despite the conflict at the pool, Dustin and Ryan did not hold a grudge. That evening during karaoke, all of the campers sang in groups. Ryan tried to sing a solo but it wasn't going well, so a few of the other boys, including Dustin, went up and sang with him. It seemed like their altercation had been temporarily resolved.

The next day we went to a nearby lake for a hike. On the bus ride back, Sasha sat with me and told me that she felt guilty for making Dustin feel sad. The other boys told her that she was the only girl Dustin wanted, and that he regarded her as the only decent girl. Then she asked me what decent meant. She decided to go to the dance with Ryan instead of Dustin because Dustin was mean and swore. On the other hand, she said that Ryan was "a gentleman and doesn't care how I look on the outside, which is important because I am overweight, and most guys don't accept that." Yet, before dinner, she told Ryan that she did not want to go to the dance with him after all. She explained that he was annoying her, and she needed space. Ryan cried and sat by a tree alone. At dinner, Sasha asked Charlie to the dance, and he said yes. Both Dustin and Ryan were dejected about Sasha and the dance.

On the night of the dance, all the campers got dressed up and went to the gym where the counselors had set up balloons and decorations. The gym was dark, and they played a lot of contemporary pop songs and two slow dances. During the first slow dance, quite a few of them partnered up, including Ray and Sarah, Mandy and Jacob, and Sasha and Charlie. The campers seemed to enjoy themselves, although the anticipation leading up to the dance was far more exciting that the dance itself. In comparison to the high drama of the first dance, the subsequent camp dances were more relaxed, with the campers abandoning the notion of needing dates for the dance.

Making friends, developing crushes, and dealing with the highs and lows of short-lived preadolescent romance are all normal parts of growing up. One benefit of the weight loss camp was that children, like Sasha, who felt excluded and rejected in their regular lives, had an opportunity to be normal. The only attention that Sasha received from her male peers at school was being teased. At camp, she had her pick of the middle school boys. The camp also offered the social rituals of youth to those who would not have felt comfortable attending a school dance. For example, Jasmine opted not to attend her homecoming dance because she could not find a dress that fit. Camp provided a place for these young people to feel accepted and to be full participants in social life.

Given these positive outcomes, weight loss camps may provide valuable social support, especially to young people who struggle with self-esteem and face exclusion or peer victimization at school. The main benefit of the weight loss camp, then, was to provide a significant source of peer acceptance among children who shared the same stigmatized identity. Being around similar others resulted in a more positive self-image and a sense of belonging.

However, because the camp focused on weight loss and not fat acceptance, the camp's impact on self-image extended beyond providing a space for bonding and self-esteem enhancement. The campers tied their changed personalities and increased confidence not only to the camp environment but also to the weight loss process and their imagined future selves. When talking about weight loss, the emotion that most commonly came up was happiness. Bridget said that losing weight made her feel good about herself. She said, "When I lose a pound, I'm really happy." Mandy wanted to lose weight because "I feel better when I'm losing weight. I'm happier and stuff." Faith said, "I would be really happy because it has been my goal for half a year now. I already lost pounds so I feel really good about myself, and I'm not expanding." Ray wanted to lose weight because it would "help me socially. I'll look good, I'll feel good. I'll be able to do stuff." The camp provided a place for the children to be socially accepted at present, but it was built around the promise of self-transformation. Campers bonded over the shared desire to be different in the future. While they enjoyed their camp identities and friendships, they saw them as time limited. Their future, postcamp selves would be thinner and happier, and weight loss was perceived as the mechanism that would make that happen.

Body Image

Body image is a form of subjective, internalized embodied inequality, the cultural system in place that ranks bodies based on their appearance. Simply put, positive body image reflects self-worth, whereas negative body image reflects a spoiled identity. Unlike conceptualizations that treat body image as a generalized, consistent state or attitude, a symbolic interactionist approach recognizes that the way people view their bodies is an active, ongoing interpretive process that depends on how people define and interpret situations and interactions.

Nearly all the campers had negative thoughts about their bodies prior to camp. Kelly regarded her own appearance with feelings ranging from resignation to disgust. She said, "Most days it was pretty negative. It was kind of like well, this is how you're going to school. You don't look good in this at all. The other thing is that I cannot stare at myself in the mirror. It creeps me out to be staring at myself and look at my body. It grosses me out. I've never liked it. And I mean, when I get out of the shower with my towel, I have my back turned to the mirror. I can't stand it at all." Kelly said that if she lost weight,

I just think that it would change so much for me if I wasn't focusing on how much I weighed every time I sat down, trying to cover up my stomach. I feel like I'd be a lot happier if I wasn't worrying about that stuff every single day and what people thought of me. I'm so self-conscious of that person standing to the left of me. What do they see from the side? Or if in these jeans, oh my gosh, my thighs are so huge when I sit down. I just think it would be so much better if I didn't have to worry about it. If I wasn't thinking about that stuff. If I actually felt good going into school wearing something instead of oh my gosh how many people can I hide from today?

Sasha also tried to conceal her body. She said, "I didn't feel right about it. I'm like this doesn't look right to me. Why am I like this? It's all my fault. I gained 20 pounds when I was in 5th grade. When I was going into 6th grade, I cried. I was so upset. I cried so much. I was upset. I wear a lot of baggy T-shirts because it hides a lot of, all my body." While they felt more outgoing at camp, they also believed that they would only have the right or ability to transfer that confidence to the world outside of camp if they became thin. The girls, especially, felt like they had to hide because they would otherwise stand out from other girls due to being bigger or the biggest.

A few of the campers rejected themselves due to their weight. Jasmine said, "Sometimes I even wish I was a different person. The first day of school, nobody would know me, and people probably wouldn't pay attention to me at all." Janet said,

> I am not a very confident person, I guess. I'm not a person with high self-esteem. I don't really care about my body. . . . I don't mean it doesn't matter how I look. I mean, I don't care about my well-being that much. . . . Personally, I seriously, seriously dislike the way I look. Yeah. And I don't know. I get stuck in I hate everything, I hate my body, I hate the way things are. I've never really been the type that's just like why don't I kill myself. More like I'm just going to let it spiral down. I don't care. This is how it's going to go.

Janet's low self-esteem and hatred of her body caused extreme detachment regarding her body size and well-being. While she denied being suicidal, she had also given up, seemingly accepting that her body and mental health would only worsen.

One overarching theme was that the campers wanted to be normal. They believed that their weight caused increased scrutiny, and they would feel better if they lost weight because their bodies would no longer draw negative attention. Ultimately, many believed that changing their body would change their personality and even their entire life. Melissa broke down in tears as she described how she felt about her body before camp. She said, "I don't really like myself because I'm this way. So I really want to get to a good weight because I just want to be at a good size and do things, what other people do. . . . I want to be thin for 8th grade. I just don't want to be so fat. I want to be like everybody else. I want to be really small." Ryan said his weight loss goal was to not stick out at either end of the weight spectrum. He said, "The people in my classroom, I'm not going to be the lightest person there. I don't want to be the heaviest person there, either. I want to be more or less normal." Likewise, Sharon said, "I don't really like being that girl who stands out in the group of friends as the bigger girl, you know. I just don't like that feeling. It makes me feel really bad about myself."

Many youth were not only concerned about losing weight but also had fear that they would be unable to stop weight gain. Mandy did not like her body before camp, particularly that when she "went on the scale the numbers would just keep rising and rising and rising." This sense of weight spiraling out of control led some campers to worry about their future selves. Jenny wanted to lose weight because she projected into the future and did not want to suffer from negative body image in high school. She said, "I want to be able to eat right, and I want to lose weight because I don't want to have to feel like oh, I'm so overweight. I can't do anything. It would make me think maybe I should lose weight because let's say three years ago I was not this badly overweight."

There were also gender differences in how the male and female campers talked about weight loss goals. The boys were more likely to say that they did not mind being bigger than other boys; they simply did not want to be quite as big as they currently were. The boys spoke more concretely of specific weights they wanted to attain—weights that would still categorize them as overweight or obese. For example, Zach wanted to go from 250 to 225 pounds, and Ray wanted to maintain a weight of 250 pounds. They all wanted to gain muscle. Tom, who was 290 pounds at the start of camp, said, "I like the way I am. I don't really wish I could be any other way. If it were up to me, I like being big. I want to lose some weight. If I'm at 250, I'd love it if I was at 250. And I'd be perfectly fine with everything." The boys were also more likely to say that they wanted to lose weight from specific areas of the body, namely their stomach and thighs, rather than overall weight loss or becoming thin.

The female campers expressed a mixture of self-acceptance and desire to lose weight, but they had more ambitious weight loss goals and higher expectations for what weight loss would do for them. Although Kyra said that she loved herself, felt pretty good about her body, and did not get bullied about her weight, she explained, "I guess I'm kind of paranoid that people are talking about my weight or talking about me. I want to stop being so self-conscious." Bridget said, "I wasn't insecure about my body, but it kind of bothers me when we have to change in gym. Everyone else is really skinny, and then I am bigger than everyone."

Jenny said that she had always liked her body and that she did not "want to be one of those super skinny girls, but I don't want to be really big. I'm kind of happy with the way I am right now. . . . Other people can make their assumptions, but I want to be happy with myself. And if I want to be overweight I can be overweight, but I shouldn't care what other people want me to be." Yet she also said that her weight prevents her from running as many laps around the gym as she used to. She said, "I want to be able to do more. I know it'll kind of sound like I care what other people think, but I would wear a dress one day and then I'd wear sweat pants the next because I'd feel like it. It makes me feel like I should have worn something better." The importance of self-acceptance was in direct dialogue with recognizing the system of embodied inequality and that others made negative judgments about her weight. Although she wanted to prioritize her own views, Jenny's weight made her feel increased appearance pressure, and she felt like she could not dress casually without playing into the "sloppy, fat woman" stereotype.

Girls engaged more explicitly in a discursive battle between self-acceptance and insecurity. On the one hand, they wanted to reject the idea that their body image was based on the harsh, negative judgments of others while concurrently feeling like they did care about how others evaluated them. While all the campers criticized their body in some way, there was also a pattern of campers who expressed both positive and negative opinions.

Female campers also had to negotiate body image when their thin friends and siblings brought up their own body weight. The campers reported feeling bad when these thin people referred to themselves as fat. "Fat talk" is the every-day talk about bodies and fatness centered on critiquing one's own body size and fatness.[1] Studies show that women who overhear fat talk are more likely to engage in fat talk themselves, and this behavior is associated with more body shame and dissatisfaction.[2] Fat talk is so normative that respondents reported being more surprised to hear positive body talk than negative body talk.[3] Body dissatisfaction and the internalization of the thin ideal, but not body weight, were associated with higher frequency of fat talk.[4]

The female campers were especially sensitive to fat talk among their thin friends. Mandy explained, "When I told my best friend that I was going to the camp, and she said, 'Oh maybe I should go because I'm fat.' When people who are really skinny say that they need to lose weight, that's pretty much the only time I put myself down and compare myself to other people."

Part of the fat talk conversational ritual is for other people to refute when someone says they are fat. Several campers noted that this was the case with their friends. Bridget said, "My friend who is heavier always says she's fat, and I always say no you're not. I'm bigger than you and she is like, no you're not. It's just back and forth." Likewise, Kelly told me what happens if she tells her friends that she feels fat:

If I do, they're always like, "Oh Kelly, stop it, you're fine. You're not overweight. You shouldn't be saying stuff like that." But it's hard when your friend is a size 2 and she's telling you that you should stop saying stuff about yourself. I hate it when my friends tell me that they think they're fat. I know I'm the exact same way. I just don't verbally say it. We'll be sitting there having a sweet, a treat, and they'll be like, "Oh my god I shouldn't be eating this. I'm so fat." It's like why do you need to say that? It makes no sense. It annoys me so much. It makes me upset. But when I think about it, I'm the exact same way.

When Kelly shared her self-criticism with others, they rejected it. She disliked it when her friends said that they were fat, particularly when they were eating certain foods. Yet she also resented that her friends, who are much slimmer than she is, denied her assessment that her body was fat.

Body Image at Camp

Jenny said that attending camp changed how she thought about herself because "sometimes you feel like you're the only one who is overweight. And then knowing that there's other people here for the same reason. It's not like I'm going to Camp Jay where everyone else is a stick." Sasha explained, "Everyone understands you here. Everyone has the same problem as you here. You don't get bullied. You don't get called fat because everyone's here for that reason, that you're overweight."

At camp, girls were able to redefine standards for femininity. The norms were different when they were in a setting where their body size was not viewed as abnormal, and being sweaty and not wearing makeup were acceptable. Kelly talked about the difference in beauty standards that had been collectively established at camp: "Hair and makeup wise, I do that every single day at home and here we do it like once a week." A higher level of comfort and feelings of acceptance at camp were common. Still, some girls reported comparing themselves to other campers, especially at the beginning of camp. Ada said, "I really didn't want to change in the cabin with a bunch of other people with me. It's just like trying to see how big she is. Is she bigger than me? This is how big she is. Does she have stretch marks? She doesn't have stretch marks. Do I have any? I don't have any stretch marks. I don't have any zits, either. I'm all like, yeah it's kind of cool. Everyone's complaining about stretch marks. Now, I'm just changing in the cabin." While Ada was initially hesitant to change in the cabin and evaluated others' bodily flaws in comparison to her own, she soon grew comfortable and felt solidarity in that everyone was complaining about their body issues. As campers lost weight, they also shared clothes to gauge their progress. Kyra said, "I didn't bring any skinny jeans to camp. One of the girls brought a pair, and I tried them on, and they didn't fit. But another girl tried them on, and they fit perfectly." While some of the appearance pressure of the outside world lessened, social comparison based on clothing sizes persisted at camp.

Dana was particularly curious about what motivated the counselors to work at a weight loss camp. She explained, "We always have counselors come who are in really good shape, and you know Matt's a college track runner and Jackie is the star of her hockey team and all of this. Then they're like 'Oh, you're here because you're overweight and I'm not.'" Further, she recounted a conversation she had with one of the counselors: "And Taylor said to me one of these years that she's been here, you know, I just want to help because it's never a problem that I've had. I've never had to think about my weight at all. And I was just like, why are you here? This makes you totally unrelatable. It's a difficult thing to deal with, and people don't understand that it's something that you have to think about all the time." Dana took issue with how Taylor had never self-problematized because she was able to manage her weight effortlessly. She resented that Taylor could not comprehend how challenging and time consuming weight loss is.

I asked Dana what she thought about Andrea, the one counselor who was overweight, and she said,

> It did feel more relatable to me. Because one year, we had one counselor who wasn't, you know, terribly overweight but she was a little bit, and she said, "I wanted to do something to lose weight this summer and so I thought why not be a counselor at a weight management camp?" And that same year we had Taylor and this woman named Amy, and they were both like in sororities, they were really pretty, they were in amazing shape. They had pictures of themselves on their Facebook in their bathing suits, which is something we would never have done. It was a lot easier to relate to the other counselor than to these women who seemed like they had perfect lives.

Although Dana did not necessarily aspire to be like Taylor and Amy, it was clear to her that their lives matched cultural notions of traditional femininity: pretty, thin, popular, sorority girls. While Dana would never publicly post a picture of herself in a bathing suit, these counselors did and were seemingly unaware of their thin privilege despite working at a weight loss camp.

It was ironic, then, that the counselor who Dana perceived as the least empathetic was the one who ran a body image workshop. Once a week, Chris and Taylor ran a program called Operation Beauty. They told the campers that even though society views beauty in one way, beauty is not based on a number or appearance. Taylor started the first session asking, "What is beauty?"

"Personality," Ada said.

"What's inside, their heart. How someone is. For some people, it is the outside: smile, face, long hair." Sasha said

"It is the way you think about yourself. If you are outgoing or shy." Jenny said.

Then they proceeded to list physical attributes associated with beauty, such as cute clothes, skinny, tan, makeup and money, body physique, six-pack abs, pretty eyes, tall.

Taylor asked, "Did you ever know someone who is beautiful but has a terrible personality?" Sasha said that there is a girl at school who was really pretty but mean on the inside, yet the boys did not care. Sasha identified embodied inequality when she saw that her classmate could be mean to others, yet her beauty still made her popular with boys. Taylor tried to direct the conversation toward valuing personality characteristics rather than outward appearance. Yet the girls were well aware of the criteria for outer beauty and the fact that personality did not overpower the social value of beauty.

Mandy brought up the traditional standard of beauty. She said, "Yeah, models and Barbie and stuff like that. They're all tiny, and have like the perfect straight hair that they don't have to do anything with, and it's just perfect. I try to tell people when they see pictures that pretty much all of it is Photoshopped. Like their face, they could have pimples, they just Photoshop them out. Girls grow up with that. Their little sisters have Barbie dolls, and from the beginning, oh that's what a girl should look like." Mandy displayed an astute critical eye toward media portrayals of flawless beauty and even attempted to educate others about the digital enhancement that models undergo. Yet she used words like "tiny" and "perfect," which were commonly used at camp to describe the popular girls at school.

Jenny said, "You don't have to be skinny to be pretty. But they should know if you're skinny, and someone says, 'Oh, you look fat,' you're not going to think anything of it. But if you are bigger and someone says that, it does hurt. It doesn't just blow over in one day." While Jenny resisted the idea that attractiveness must be tied to a thin body, she also perceived thin people as being protected from emotional harm because it would not resonate with them if they are called fat. Jenny noted that even if one accepts alternative definitions of beauty, fat stigma still hurts.

Taylor wrote Self-Affirmation on the board. She handed out a piece of paper and told each girl to write down things that she is good at and how her body helps her to do those things. Then we all read them aloud. She explained that self-affirmation is promoting integrity through recognizing your strengths. The focus was on "positive talents that your body lets you do even if you are having a bad hair day." Then Taylor brought up fat talk and said, "Fat talk free is the way to be." She asked for examples of fat talk.

"At one dance, girls in the corner were standing there saying 'I look fat in this dress,'" Ada said.

"A super skinny girl said that she was so fat and needed to lose 5 pounds," Jenny said.

"My friend is tiny and says, Oh, I'm so fat," Bridget said.

"America's need to be thin makes us feel negative," Taylor replied.

While she acknowledged the existence and negative impact of fat talk, Taylor did not address strategies for dealing with it. She then handed out a piece of paper and told them to write down things they hate about their body. Ada said, "Oh, this one is easy." Faith asked if we had to read it out loud because she did not want to. Several of them said they hated fitting into their parent's clothes. Jenny could not fit into her older sister's clothes, but she could fit into her mom's. Sasha agreed, saying that she could fit into her dad's but not her mom's clothes. Not surprising, the campers brought up concerns related to body size, especially fitting into adult-sized clothes as a child. Once again, the camp offered the children a place to share their body image concerns with sympathetic others, but it did little to promote size acceptance, even during a body image workshop.

The Camp Odyssey Success Story

Dana's story illustrates the pivotal role that Camp Odyssey had in shaping her view on her past, present, and future selves. When Dana began attending camp at age 11, she was 30 pounds heavier and she had been up to 50 pounds heavier than she was at present. Despite her weight, she described a "true" self that was athletic. Comparing herself to another camper made her recognize that she should transform her postcamp self and work out year round.

> Two years ago, Kristy came at about the same weight that I was, and that was like, I don't know, something really high, like 220. It was not good, and we're the same height. So we were very, very similar. We looked similar, and everyone thought we were the same person. And then we both lost quite a bit of weight, and then we both kind of stayed active the next year. But she joined rowing, and she lost a ton of weight. She just dropped. And then she came back and she was in really good shape, and I was like this is ridiculous. Why didn't I do that? Why haven't I done that? I need to do that right now. So this past year, I work out every day. I get up at 5:30 in the morning, and I go to the gym before school because I have an after school job so I don't have time then. I made the decision. I said this is gross. I don't want to be that person anymore.

For Dana, seeing a fellow camper lose weight through increased physical activity inspired her to change her behavior. The frustration and disgust that she felt when she did not lose as much weight as her camp friend with whom she had so much in common had a powerful impact on her sense of self. She made the decision to change her behavior because she wanted to be a different type of person. In addition to the peer comparison with someone who had been similar to her at one time and then changed, the camp also provided a role model in the form of a counselor who was a medical student with a busy schedule. This counselor told them that you make time to exercise no matter what else is going on. She said that stuck with her, and she rearranged everything so that she would have time to work out.

Dana rejected her past self who did not work out daily because she did not see herself as

> the kind of person who is lazy and unmotivated and doesn't do things. I like being strong and athletic. That's part of why I come to camp, when I come here, I am the most athletic person. When we play soccer, I'm against the counselors and I win races. I don't think that I'm supposed to be a lazy person. The person I am should be someone who is more athletic and more able to do things. And so, this last year, I was just like, this is ridiculous. I am the kind of person who would work out every day, so I'm just going to do it.

Dana talked about her future self as who she is "supposed to be" and "meant" to be. For her, the body she had did not match her true inner self, which was a disciplined athlete. It was not the passive internalization of camp messages about exercise and nutrition that transformed Dana. Rather, it was the interactional process of seeing other people enact and reinforce the camp's messages that motivated her to change her behavior and her self-concept outside of camp. The camp provided not only supportive others but also inspirational motivators.

After five summers with Camp Odyssey, Dana was regarded as a success story and role model by the camp directors and staff. Dana lost weight and became the type of person who believed in and enacted self-control, discipline, and athleticism, which were the hallmarks of the Camp Odyssey discourse. However, Dana was a rare exception. Most other campers were not able to make the self and bodily transformation as effectively as she did.

The Dark Side of Camp Odyssey

Dana and Sharon were both 16-year-old junior counselors who were heralded as role models. Sharon had attended Camp Odyssey twice before. While camp provided a space of comfort for those who wanted to change their bodies, it also reinforced their stigmatized identity. Like many others, Sharon explained that she attended camp because it made her feel better about herself.

> I find that every time that I come to camp, I go back home so much happier and more confident with myself. I'm always a lot more confident, which is why I wanted to come here. Because my past year has been really, really bad, and I lost a lot of confidence in myself. So I came here and I'm hoping I go home a lot more happy and more confident. Because it used to do that. I'm just generally a really shy person. I feel like I fit in more here. When I come back from camp, I feel a lot happier with my body and more outgoing.

Sharon linked her camp experiences to positive outcomes, and she was motivated to return to camp because she craved feeling like that again after a difficult year. Yet, unlike Dana, Sharon did not conform to Camp Odyssey's messages about self-transformation and weight loss. In fact, she felt like she did not belong at camp this summer because she had suffered from an eating disorder for the past year. She said, "I feel like I shouldn't be here. Because they'll think I've lost weight in a healthy way, but I haven't at all." Sharon was bulimic. She said, "I felt good because I could eat a whole bunch and then not feel full. I could eat all this food and then throw it all up and I felt ok." Rather than managing her fullness using camp-sanctioned methods like the hunger scale, Sharon found an alternative way to eat what she wanted without being too full or gaining weight.

Sharon's eating disorder was likely caused by a number of factors. Her sister had struggled with anorexia in the past, her parent's relationship was strained, and she had a difficult dynamic with her mother. When her boyfriend cheated on her with one of her close friends, Sharon's self-esteem was shattered, which exacerbated her poor body image and made bulimia appealing. In my interview with her, I asked whether she thought that attending a weight loss camp contributed to her eating disorder.

> I've just always been that bigger person, and I think I got older and started hearing more about these eating disorders. I went to this weight loss camp. I felt kind of like, I don't know how to describe it, out of place. Whenever I would think, I'm fat. I would always think the reason, the way to prove I'm fat is that I went to a fat camp. I'm obviously fat. There's no way of telling me that I'm not because I went to a camp. I'm overweight. I need to lose weight. It's just like I couldn't do it any other way. So I think that [bulimia] did the trick a little bit.

The camp did not directly cause Sharon's eating disorder, and she was aware that her new method of weight management would be met with disapproval by the camp leadership if they knew. At the same time, in her mind, being a weight loss camper confirmed that she was fat. By virtue of participation, Sharon internalized that her body size was viewed as a problem in need of treatment. Attending a weight loss camp can reinforce the identity of being "obese" even if the intent is bodily change and stigma exit to a thin identity.

Sharon's story points to the idea that naming the problem and validating it as needing intervention leads to internalization. Under the right circumstances, intensive attention to dieting, exercise, and body concerns can cause disordered eating. Many young people, Sharon included, viewed camp as a boost to their self-esteem. However, this weight loss environment also validated the message that they had a problematic body and that they must change themselves in order to be happy outside of camp. Sharon's story reveals that weight loss programs can instill a dieting mentality and potentially lead to eating disorders. Weight loss programs, including Camp Odyssey, send mixed messages that promote both self-acceptance and body change. The camp's intent was to produce embodied and internalized self-change that led to a healthier lifestyle, as in Dana's story. Unfortunately, those messages can also lead to problematic coping strategies, such as eating disorders.

Discussion

What should we make of the fact that the children liked attending a weight loss camp? On the positive side, the campers experienced social benefits, such as feeling accepted and normal, having fun, participating in summer camp activities, making friends, and developing flirtations. For those who were seeking to change their eating and exercise habits, the camp provided an enormous amount of educational material and role models that could potentially influence the camper's long-term behavior and body size, as was the case with Dana. On the other hand, those very same messages about self-control, managing fullness, and problematizing the fat body could also potentially aggravate poor body image and disordered eating, as was the case with Sharon.

Beyond the cautionary tale of weight management practices that led to a full-fledged eating disorder, the camp also amplified the ambivalent and contradictory cultural beliefs of positive body image and bodily change. In the span of two hours, the campers were exposed to messages about changing habits and self-control and then went straight to a body image workshop where they were told to love their bodies and to be critical of the media's unrealistic standards of beauty. The campers were told to reject their self-consciousness about being fat, yet they should still work to remove fat from their bodies so that they can feel less self-conscious. These messages were reflected in my interviews with the campers, who expressed both self-acceptance and self-criticism, sometimes within the same sentences.

While the camp at least made the attempt to address body image issues and fat stigma, the reality was that the camp's main aim was to get the children to change their habits and bodies. By sending the message that they should love themselves and change themselves, the children were exposed to conflicting messages about body image. I argue that these messages are just as psychologically harmful as overt fat shaming, and perhaps even more so, because they are complex and insidious. By pairing the fun of camp, the temporary self-esteem boost of peer acceptance and weight loss, and paying lip service to body acceptance along with strong messages about the importance of body transformation, the children internalized antifat discourse and further problematized fatness. The camp was able to strongly influence the children's beliefs about fatness, weight loss, and their sense of self precisely because the shaming and stigmatizing messages were sugarcoated with messages of empowerment, acceptance, and positive emotional experiences. While the weight loss that occurred at camp was likely to be short term, the effects of validating anti-fat views through temporary experiential pleasures and promoting weight loss as the key to happiness were likely to be far more long lasting.

8

Conclusion

During the last few days of camp, the children were tired and irritable. After nearly a month of being away from their home, they looked forward to being back with their family and sleeping in their own bed. The main topic of conversation during those last days was what it would be like to maintain their weight loss at home. Sharon and Dana, the junior counselors, led a session on returning home. Although this topic had been covered many times, the campers still asked questions. Dana told them, "Your first night back is weird. Your clothes are too big. It is weird to eat because you are thrown into making choices. It is like Visitors Day every day. There is no one to answer to. You are really by yourself. You are used to having twenty-five people for support, but you have to learn self-reliance. It is up to you. If you want it, you have to try. Everyone will expect you to eat more. They will be surprised by how little you eat." The campers were told that transitioning from camp life to regular life would feel different—even their clothes would feel strange on their new body. The biggest key to success when facing pressure from friends and family to go back to old habits was self-control. The camp support structure (and social control) would be gone, so it was entirely up to the child to maintain self-control despite the temptations and expectations of their old environment.

When Taylor, a counselor, asked about family members sabotaging their child's change in habits, Sharon said that others pressured her to eat more and "people asked what was wrong with me. You come back a new person, so they are confused. But they get used it. I changed, but they got used to it." While the campers had undergone a month of intensive self-change, they were returning to a world where people still knew them as their former self who had precamp habits. Sharon assured the campers that people would adjust to these changes if the campers stayed firm with their new ways of being.

Dana warned that the campers could lose their new habits and gain weight if they did not create a healthy routine at home and stick with it. She said, "I have been to camp five times. Sometimes I did not follow up with what I learned at camp at all. I felt good after camp. So I thought, why would I let this happen? Why feel like crap again? I came back to camp to relearn and decided to make the changes at home for good."

All the returning campers reported backsliding and regaining the weight they had lost at camp. Dana was able to make the adjustments at home only after several years at camp. The typical story of what happened after camp was captured by Ray. He said, "Last year, after camp, I had a lot of high hopes and expectations. By September, I really felt that it might not happen, and then by December, thinking about camp and camp-related stuff was gone."

Embodied Inequality

My interest in studying a weight loss camp was not to determine how effective it was as a weight loss program. Rather, I was interested in how it served as a location for children to negotiate discourses about body-size inequality through social interactions. Embodied inequality is entrenched in the pervasive antiobesity discourse that children encounter from their peers, schools, doctors, and the media. The weight loss camp reinforced the internalization of bodily inadequacy and problematization. In this book, I used ethnographic and interview data to explore *processes* of embodied inequality: how the children came to recognize inequalities related to their body size, how they explained the causes of those differences, and how they responded to microlevel injustices in their lives. Embodied inequality is constructed and negotiated through interactional processes, including resocialization, social comparisons, and attribution.

Children learned to problematize their bodies through interactions with their peers prior to attending camp. Gender was an important dimension in crafting the children's understandings of how bodies played a role in the status systems of their peer groups. Girls placed greater emotional emphasis on appearance, especially clothing, whereas boys noticed their lower status through their inability to excel at athletics. After failed attempts at losing weight with family members, many of the children and their families sought enrollment at a weight loss camp as a means of stigma management. Yet participating in such a program also raised the specter that their peers would stigmatize them for attending a "fat camp." By concealing their participation or reframing the camp as a fitness or weight management camp, the children were able to preserve their self-image. This framing also allowed for normal or slightly overweight children to participate since they were seeking improved health and fitness, which was ostensibly the purpose of the camp.

At Camp Odyssey, the program engaged children in a body project and taught them new skills, knowledge, and habits related to nutrition, portion size, and physical activity. The program also provided an environment for children to reset the connection between their mind and body. Techniques aimed at getting children to recalibrate their hunger and use a different style of eating moved beyond the realm of intentional and strategic action to include embodied change. In addition to these resocialization processes, social control mechanisms and an immersive environment at camp supported resocialization and weight loss in the short term. Indeed, all campers lost weight. However, the long-term effectiveness of the camp's resocialization efforts is unlikely as evidenced by their brief encounters with the outside world during camp. When the children left camp for a water park excursion, it was clear that many could identify features of resocialization in a camp-sanctioned narrative, but they found it difficult to enact these changes without the support and control of the camp. As the camp staff acknowledged, camp was not a "magic bullet." In order for weight loss to be maintained or continued, the resocialization process would have to be adopted by the home environment. The children may have acquired knowledge, achieved physical changes, and experienced a new way of being, but this was unlikely to be sustained without adults who continue the camp's resocialization techniques at home.

The Camp Odyssey staff and directors did not engage in coercive or overtly shaming tactics. Daily interactions were positive, and the children had fun. In fact, the children pointed to a number of psychological benefits to the friendships they made at camp. Many of the campers felt bullied and insecure at school, so camp was a welcome social environment where they could relate to and be accepted by others. These positive aspects of camp suggest that children who struggle with body image benefit from being around similar others. At the same time, the camp conveyed powerful messages about self-control, character, morality, and the values of "healthism," which equated self-worth to body size. These covert methods of shame and self-control motivated the children to lose weight, but the methods also damaged their self-worth and reinforced antifat attitudes. Additionally, the high failure rate of dieting in general, and the short-term nature of camp, created a situation where some children absorbed the values of camp but could not successfully implement the camp's plan when they returned home. Unable to lose weight without the social control of camp, some campers blamed themselves for not maintaining their camp weight loss, and a few developed eating disorders.

The children held multiple explanations for what causes obesity, and these ideas were shaped by the dynamic interactive process of attending a weight loss camp. Some campers attributed body weight to biological and genetic components and used this to explain why losing weight is more difficult for some people than others. From the camp's perspective, attributing body weight to biological causes rather than effort and self-control was incorrect. The camp used a number of strategies to defuse the attribution that some people lacked the ability to be thin. The children were taught to use strategies to change their thought patterns and to cultivate new habits. Despite the children's hope that what they learned at camp would transform their body, they also brought their previous experiences and observations with them, including the idea that body size is a matter of luck. The concept of "luck" reflects a sense of embodied inequality given that some people have thinner bodies without expending effort or making sacrifices like those who are overweight.

Children and the Pursuit of Weight Loss

What is in a child's best interest if he or she is heavier than other children? Given the negative social consequences of discrimination and mistreatment, some might say that the proper agentic response to embodied inequality would be to lose weight. The little girl who loses 30 pounds may very well be more accepted by others. People must deal with the culture they encounter presently and make the best choices they can. Many of the children at the weight loss camp suffered tremendously due to their weight, and it is not hard to understand why they sought a solution to the problems they faced. Adults may wish to protect children from suffering and harm, but we must also question whether children's weight loss programs do more harm than good. The possible benefits of weight loss must be evaluated against the psychological consequences (e.g., poor body image, eating disorders) of focusing on weight at such a young age.

First, even if weight loss is encouraged to manage certain health conditions, it is unlikely that the weight lost will be permanent for the majority of children who attempt to become thinner. Based on my observations and a growing body of research, it is clear that body weight is not simply a result of excess calories, eating style, and physical activity.[1] While those factors play a role, much remains unanswered regarding why some people gain weight and others do not, despite similar lifestyles. This points to the limitations of individual-level blame and invites questioning the larger food system that is in place. One intriguing theory is that the rise in childhood obesity may be linked to environmental toxins, particularly endocrine-disrupting chemicals.[2] Yet, regardless of how systemic or multifaceted the cause of obesity truly is, the camp staff viewed weight as a matter of personal responsibility, and the children at the camp were seeking individual-level solutions. When the focus is on calorie counting, self-control, and healthism, the stigmatization of obesity persists while more systemic explanations and solutions are ignored. As school and community education programs about health, nutrition, fitness, and obesity become more common, future research should examine the short-term and long-term effects of these resocialization attempts on self-esteem and body size.

The most concerning aspect of resocialization at the weight loss camp is that, rather than instilling healthy habits, the experience may have unintentionally set up the children to become lifelong cyclical dieters. While removing the children from their families was effective as a short-term solution, the children were likely to regain the weight upon their return home. This inadvertent yo-yo model of weight management is an unhealthy precedent to set. Research suggests that losing and gaining weight may cause more health problems than being overweight.[3] Moralistic undertones and contradictory messages about weight management are unfair to all dieters, but these are particularly burdensome for children. The camp continually told children to work on self-control when, in fact, their weight loss was due in large part to the social control of the camp environment. By teaching children to equate health with morality and self-control with self-esteem, the camp sent the message to children that the pursuit of dieting was a valuable—and value-laden—personality trait. Most troubling of all was the unfair expectation that children maintain the changes on their own at home while also teaching their adult family members how to lose weight.

Weight loss programs for children reflect a number of disturbing cultural components. First, the act of endorsing children's weight loss reinforces the fact that to be successful you need to be thin. Conflating success and happiness with body size means that there is little space for overweight people to be associated with those positive attributes. Antifat culture conveys the message to children that who they are and how much they are worth depend on what their body weighs, how they look, and what they can do physically. When self-worth is tied to what bodies do and look like then it is entirely based on how society values certain bodies over others. The logic that high self-esteem is necessary to be happy and successful, and in order to have self-esteem one must be thin or become thin through weight loss efforts, creates psychological damage for children. The camp sent the message that feeling confident is based on feeling good about your body, and more importantly, feeling good is tied to having control over what your body looks like and weighs.

The children themselves felt that being overweight was unhealthy and socially stigmatized. They viewed the weight loss camp as an agentic solution to change their past eating and exercise habits so that they could feel better about themselves and fit in. Unfortunately, the "success" of the camp in providing short-term weight loss and a self-esteem boost may have actually been its ultimate downfall. If the benefits of that environment cannot be transferred and sustained in the outside world, the children were not actually resocialized in terms of eating and exercise habits. Instead, the camp reinforced and magnified the cultural beliefs that problematized their weight. The children received clear messages that being a good person and self-esteem were linked to pursuing weight loss.

Second, an increasing emphasis on continual self-change and self-improvement ultimately undermines the self-esteem that it is meant to create. What are we really teaching our children when we make childhood obesity a social evil and regard fatness as a failure? We teach children that they must change themselves—through consuming products and services to make them thinner and to use feelings of inadequacy to motivate a change of habits. If successful, the child must then anxiously try to maintain any "improvements" that occur. Our fat-phobic culture is toxic for all children, not just those who are labeled as overweight or obese. All children are socialized to change rather than to accept appearance diversity and differences in ability. Conforming to body ideals may improve life for some individuals by lessening stigma and discrimination, yet the pervasive idea that the solution to human suffering or social injustice is through a harmful and endless cycle of bodily modifications comes at a far greater cost.

While wanting children to be healthy and happy is a dominant, virtually unquestioned cultural value, linking health and happiness to body size only reinforces stigma, prejudice, and inequality based on body size. The undue emotional burden of requiring thinness, health, and strict control of nutrition and physical activity places a great deal of stress on the youngest members of society. Promoting antiobesity initiatives that link social problems to children's bodies serves to shame and demean people and reinforces expectations that self-esteem and happiness are tied to physical bodies.

Fat Acceptance for Children

While I believe that most people are sympathetic to the plight of children who struggle with their body image and self-esteem, is fat acceptance for children possible? Most people have never heard of or do not support the fat acceptance movement for adults, so the idea that people will embrace fat acceptance for children is highly unlikely at the present time. The fat acceptance movement consists of mostly very large, white women. In reading their stories, one discovers that most had first internalized fat negativity and body shame in their early years, then later in life decided to reject those cultural beliefs and create a counterculture. This points to the idea that resistance is a long process, one that typically does not start in childhood. Fat acceptance occurs in adulthood because the fat identity is something that has become a stable identity. An adult who has consistently been fat, perhaps since childhood or adolescence, is able to see that his or her body size is not going to change, even after repeated attempts at weight loss. If this is the case, then the options are either to be a lifelong dieter (with little probability of success or cyclical weight loss and gains) or to embrace body acceptance.

On the other hand, the way the children connect their body image to their identities is in flux. Children are in a state of becoming a self, becoming an adult, and becoming a body. As their sense of self develops, their body may lead to a fat identity, as Ada pointed out when she said that if she does not lose weight "maybe I was born this way." Alternatively, they may feel like their body does not match their inner self, and they want to change their body to conform to who they think they really are or aspire to be. The latter enforces the idea that body size is a choice, and that we select and modify our appearance and body to show the world our desired inner self.

While future selves are powerful conceptual constructs to motivate weight loss for adults, the future self is even more salient for children. They do not know yet if being fat is permanent. If they accept fatness, it may be interpreted as though they have already decided their future self and given up hope that their future self can be thin. Indeed, children's bodies are physiologically changing and growing. Weight gain is part of the growth process for children. They might grow in height or lose weight over time. Thus the possibility for a child's body to change is more likely than it is for adults, who generally gain weight as they age. In contrast, adults have more evidence that their fatness is stable and that their height will no longer change either.

Further, children are typically viewed as being only partially agentic and still under considerable influence by society and especially the family environment. A child's body size is seen, at least in part, as a matter of adult responsibility. Therefore, fat acceptance for children would likely be viewed by some as letting parents off the hook for damaging their children through unhealthy practices and putting them at risk for diseases. While obesity is often characterized in moral terms, this is especially heightened when children are involved and could be viewed as victims. This sentiment is strong enough that some children have been removed from their home due to obesity that is seen as a form of child abuse or neglect.

Finally, there are vested financial interests in perpetuating the belief that body weight is under individual control. A huge industry exists to make people believe that if they buy certain things they can become slimmer. Beautiful, healthy bodies keep people insecure so they consume and spend money for a fix. Problematizing bodies leads to spending money to fix bodies. The earlier in the life course that people problematize their body, the more money they will spend over their lifetime. Children's weight loss programs are an untapped market for the commercial diet industry.

For all these reasons, it is unlikely that there will be a broad-based fat acceptance movement for children. Yet I hope that this book provides insight into the suffering and injustice faced by young children whose bodies are problematized amid the "obesity epidemic" and that adults will be moved to confront and dismantle embodied inequality. First, all children should be taught about body size diversity and undergo antibullying workshops. Second, access to nutritious food and accessible physical activity should be available to all children. Third, for children who are concerned about their weight, being around others with similar experiences can prove comforting. Activities, teams, support groups, and, yes, even summer camps that promote Health At Every Size and body acceptance should be affordable and provided as readily as traditional athletic teams. Parents, teachers, and other adults should focus their time, attention, and energy on engaging children, especially those marginalized by body size, in developing their talents and interests in ways that can be sources of self-esteem and purpose. Rather than connecting self-esteem to body projects or self-improvement, children should be encouraged to find their own passions and connect with people who share their interests. Finally, more attention needs to be paid to the structural causes of the population's weight gain, and the moral panic over childhood obesity needs to be critiqued. Both adults and children would benefit from the elimination of antiobesity discourse.

Acknowledgments

Many people had a hand in developing this project. I am indebted to the faculty at Indiana University for their feedback during my dissertation research, and my colleagues at Florida Atlantic University who supported me as I turned my dissertation into this book during my first years as an assistant professor. Brent Harger, Lotus Seeley, and Patricia Widener provided helpful feedback on earlier versions of the book. I especially thank Ashley Ostroot for her outstanding work as my research assistant during the summer of 2017. My editor at Rutgers University Press, Peter Mickulas, as well as the three reviewers of the book, greatly improved the book. A special thank you to my friend Maria Torti for the cover concept.

Parts of chapter 5 appear in the article, "Embodied Resocialization at a Children's Weight Loss Camp," which was originally published in *Ethnography* 17, no. 4 (2016): 539–558. A version of chapter 2, "Accomplishing Empathy: An Ethnography of a Children's Weight Loss Camp," was published in *SAGE Research Methods Cases* (2018). Thanks to SAGE publications for permission to use these works in the book.

My family has been unwaveringly supportive as I spent years working on this project, moved across the country several times for academic jobs, and finally completed the book. My mother, Kimberly McGraw, and my sister, Brittany Quinn, kept me grounded and added humor to my life during each step of this journey. I also thank my partner, Brandon Miller, for reading every word of the final manuscript and being the book's biggest fan.

My Nan, Lois Backstrom, would have been so proud that I wrote a book. She always believed that I would. This book is dedicated to her.

Finally, I thank the camp directors and staff for giving me access to the camp and answering my questions along the way. Most importantly, I am grateful to the children who shared their camp experience with me. While this book portrays only a snapshot of their childhoods, I hope that it conveys the complexity, vulnerability, and honesty of their lives during that time.

Notes

Chapter 1   Embodied Inequality, Childhood Obesity, and the "Problem Child"

1 Abby Ellin, *Teenage Waistland: A Former Fat-Camper Weighs in on Living Large, Losing Weight, and How Parents Can (and Can't) Help* (New York: PublicAffairs, 2005).
2 Julie Guthman, *Weighing In: Obesity, Food Justice, and the Limits of Capitalism* (Berkeley: University of California Press, 2011).
3 Cynthia L. Ogden, "Prevalence of High Body Mass Index in U.S. Children and Adolescents, 2007–2008," *Medical Benefits* 27, no. 3 (2010): 3. Ogden found that "since 1980, the prevalence of BMI for age at or above the 95th percentile (sometimes termed 'obese') has tripled among school-age children and adolescents, and it remains high at approximately 17%."
4 Christine Halse, "Bio-Citizenship: Virtue Discourses and the Birth of the Bio-Citizen," in *Biopolitics and the 'Obesity Epidemic': Governing Bodies*, ed. Jan Wright and Valerie Harwood, 45–59 (New York: Routledge, 2009).
5 Lewis A. Barness, John. M. Opitz, and Enid Gilbert-Barness, "Obesity: Genetic, Molecular, and Environmental Aspects," *American Journal of Medical Genetics* 143A (2007): 3016–3034. Barness et al. found that childhood obesity is associated with multiple chronic illnesses, including (but not limited to) type 2 diabetes, hypertension, polycystic ovary syndrome, nonalcoholic fatty liver disease, obstructive apnea, and orthopedic complications.
6 Penny Gordon-Larsen, Natalie S. The, and Linda S. Adair, "Longitudinal Trends in Obesity in the United States from Adolescence to the Third Decade of Life," *Obesity* 18, no. 9 (2010): 1802. Gordon-Larsen et al. found that "the vast majority (90%) of obese adolescents remained obese into their 30s: 94% of females overall, 95% of black females, and 88% of males remained obese."
7 Mission: Readiness Military Leaders for Kids. "Too Fat to Fight: Retired Military Leaders Want Junk Food out of America's Schools" (2010): 1–11. http://cdn.missionreadiness.org/MR_Too_Fat_to_Fight-1.pdf.
8 *Killer at Large: Why Obesity Is America's Greatest Threat*, directed by Stephen Greenstreet (New York: Disinformation Company; Shinebox Media Productions, 2009), DVD.

9 Halse, "Bio-Citizenship."

10 Robert J. Kuczmarksi and Katherine M. Flegal, "Criteria for Definition of Overweight in Transition: Background and Recommendations for the United States," *American Journal of Clinical Nutrition* 72 (2000): 1074–1091.

11 Paul Campos, *The Obesity Myth* (New York: Gotham Books, 2004); Paul Campos, Abigail Saguy, Paul Ernsberger, Eric Oliver, and Glen Gaesser, "The Epidemiology of Overweight and Obesity: Public Health Crisis or Moral Panic?" *International Journal of Epidemiology* 35 (2006): 55–60; Katherine M. Flegal, Barry I. Graubard, David F. Williamson, and Mitchell H. Gail, "Excess Deaths Associated with Underweight, Overweight, and Obesity," *Journal of the American Medical Association* 293, no. 15 (2005): 1861–1867; Michael Gard and Jan Wright, *The Obesity Epidemic: Science, Morality, and Ideology* (New York: Routledge, 2005).

12 Campos, *Obesity Myth*.

13 Kathleen Lebesco, *Revolting Bodies: The Struggle to Redefine Fat Identity* (Boston: University of Massachusetts Press, 2004).

14 Simone Fullagar, "Governing Health Family Lifestyles through Discourses of Risk and Responsibility" in *Biopolitics and the 'Obesity Epidemic': Governing Bodies*, ed. Jan Wright and Valerie Harwood, 108–126 (New York: Routledge, 2009); Halse, "Bio-Citizenship."

15 Rachel Colls and Bethan Evans, "Embodying Responsibility: Children's Health and Supermarket Initiatives," *Environment and Planning A* 40, (2008), 615–631.

16 Abigail C. Saguy and Rene Almeling, "Fat in the Fire? Science, the News Media, and the 'Obesity Epidemic,'" *Sociological Forum* 23, no. 1 (2008): 53–83.

17 John Coveney, "The Government of Girth," *Health Sociology Review* 17, no. 2 (2008): 199–212.

18 John Coveney, *Food, Morals and Meaning: The Pleasure and Anxiety of Eating* (London: Routledge, 2006).

19 Abigail C. Saguy, *What's Wrong with Fat?* (Oxford: Oxford University Press, 2013).

20 Sarah Trainer, Alexandra Brewis, Deborah Williams, and Jose Rosales Chaves, "Obese, Fat, or 'Just Big'? Young Adult Deployment of and Reactions to Weight Terms," *Human Organization* 74, no. 3 (2015): 267.

21 Erving Goffman, *The Presentation of Self in Everyday Life* (New York: Doubleday, 1959).

22 Goffman, *Presentation of Self*.

23 Erving Goffman, *Stigma: Notes on the Management of a Spoiled Identity* (Englewood Cliffs, NJ: Prentice Hall, 1963).

24 Bruce G. Link and Jo C. Phelan, "Conceptualizing Stigma," *Annual Review of Sociology* 27 (2001): 363–385.

25 Michèle Lamont and Annette Lareau, "Cultural Capital: Allusions, Gaps and Glissandos in Recent Theoretical Developments," *Sociological Theory* 6 (1988): 153–168.

26 Abigail C. Saguy and Kjerstin Gruys, "Morality and Health: News Media Constructions of Overweight and Eating Disorders," *Social Problems* 57, no. 2 (2010): 231–250.

27 Shari L. Dworkin and Faye Linda Wachs, *Body Panic: Gender, Health, and the Selling of Fitness* (New York: New York University Press, 2009).

28 Samantha Kwan and Mary Nell Trautner, "Beauty Work: Individual and

Institutional Rewards, the Reproduction of Gender, and Questions of Agency," *Sociology Compass* 3, no. 1 (2009): 49–71.

29   Cecilia L. Ridgeway, *Framed by Gender: How Gender Inequality Persists in the Modern World* (New York: Oxford University Press, 2011); Michael Sauder, "Symbols and Contexts: An Interactionist Approach to the Study of Social Status," *Sociological Quarterly* 46, no. 2 (2005): 279–298.

30   Susan Averett and Sanders Korenman, "Black-White Differences in Social and Economic Consequences of Obesity," *International Journal of Obesity* 23, no. 2 (1999): 166–173; Christian S. Crandall and Rebecca Martinez, "Culture, Ideology, and Antifat Attitudes," *Personality and Social Psychology Bulletin* 22, no. 11 (1996): 1165–1176.

31   Rebecca M. Puhl and Kelly D. Brownell, "Bias, Discrimination, and Obesity," *Obesity Research* 9 (2001): 788–805; Rebecca M. Puhl and Kelly D. Brownell, "Psychosocial Origins of Obesity Stigma: Toward Changing a Powerful and Pervasive Bias," *Obesity Reviews* 4, no. 4 (2003): 213–227; Bethany A. Teachman, Kathrine D. Gapinski, Kelly D. Brownell, Melissa Rawlins, and Subathra Jeyaram, "Demonstrations of Implicit Anti-Fat Bias: The Impact of Providing Causal Information and Evoking Empathy," *Health Psychology* 22, no. 1 (2003): 68–78; Amy Erdman Farrell, *Fat Shame: Stigma and the Fat Body in American Culture* (New York: New York University Press, 2011); Rebecca M. Puhl and Chelsea A. Heuer, "The Stigma of Obesity: A Review and Update," *Obesity* 17, no. 5 (2009): 941–964.

32   Rebecca. M. Puhl, T. Andreyeva, and Kelly D. Brownell, "Perceptions of Weight Discrimination: Prevalence and Comparison to Race and Gender Discrimination in America," *International Journal of Obesity* 32 (2008), 992–1000; Deborah Carr and Michael A. Friedman, "Is Obesity Stigmatizing? Body Weight, Perceived Discrimination, and Psychological Well-Being in the United States," *Journal of Health and Social Behavior* 46 (2005): 244–259; Puhl and Brownell, "Bias, Discrimination, and Obesity."

33   Carr and Friedman, "Is Obesity Stigmatizing?"; John Cawley, "The Impact of Obesity on Wages," *Journal of Human Resources* 39 (2004): 451–474; Katherine M. Haskins and H. Edward Ransford, "The Relationship between Weight and Career Payoffs among Women," *Sociological Forum* 14 (1999): 295–318; Puhl and Brownell, "Bias, Discrimination, and Obesity."

34   Charles L. Baum and William F. Ford, "The Wage Effects of Obesity: A Longitudinal Study," *Health Economics* 13, no. 9 (2004): 885–899. Baum and Ford found that both men and women—but particularly women—who are obese experience persistent wage penalties over the first two decades of their careers, and that these penalties may be channeled through other variables, such as job discrimination, health-related factors, and/or obese workers' behavior; John Cawley, "The Impact of Obesity on Wages," *Journal of Human Resources* 39 (2004): 468. Cawley found that "heavier white females, black females, Hispanic females, and Hispanic males tend to earn less, and heavier black males tend to earn more than their lighter counterparts."

35   Yen-hsin Alice Cheng and Nancy S. Landale, "Adolescent Overweight, Social Relationships and the Transition to First Sex: Gender and Racial Variations," *Perspectives on Sexual and Reproductive Health* 43, no. 1 (2011): 6–15; Robert Crosnoe, "Gender, Obesity, and Education," *Sociology of Education* 80 (2007): 241–260.

36 Puhl, Andreyeva, and Brownell, "Perceptions of Weight Discrimination." Puhl et al. found that women were twice as likely as men to report discrimination due to weight/height. Types of discrimination included being treated with less respect and courtesy, being treated as inferior, being called names and/or being insulted, and receiving poorer service at restaurants.

37 Cawley, "The Impact of Obesity on Wages," 468; Katherine Mason, "The Unequal Weight of Discrimination: Gender, Body Size, and Income Inequality," *Social Problems* 59, no. 3 (2012): 411–435.

38 Janna L. Fikkan and Esther D. Rothblum, "Is Fat a Feminist Issue? Exploring the Gendered Nature of Weight Bias," *Sex Roles* 66, no. 9 (2011): 575–592. Fikkan and Rothblum argue that women are more likely to be discriminated based on their weight, and that this discrimination negatively influences a number of factors, including perceived supervisory potential, self-discipline, professional appearance, personal hygiene, ability to perform a physically strenuous job, reliability, dependability, honesty, ability to inspire, desirability as a coworker, and likelihood of being recommended for hiring. Overweight women also have lower household incomes, lower probability of marriage, and lower likelihood of employment.

39 Marika Tiggemann and Esther D. Rothblum, "Gender Differences in Social Consequences of Perceived Overweight in the United States and Australia," *Sex Roles* 18, no. 1/2 (1988): 75–86.

40 Michael A. Friedman and Kelly D. Brownell, "Psychological Correlates of Obesity: Moving to the Next Research Generation," *Psychological Bulletin* 117, no. 1 (1995): 3–20.

41 Carr and Friedman, "Is Obesity Stigmatizing?"

42 Ibid.

43 Markus H. Schafer and Kenneth F. Ferraro, "The Stigma of Obesity: Does Perceived Weight Discrimination Affect Identity and Physical Health?" *Social Psychology Quarterly* 74, no. 1 (2011): 76–97.

44 Jane Wardle and Lucy Cooke, "The Impact of Obesity on Psychological Well-being," *Best Practice & Research Clinical Endocrinology & Metabolism* 19, no. 3 (2005): 421–440.

45 Jennifer A. Harriger, Rachel M. Calogero, David. C. Witherington, and Jane Ellen Smith, "Body Size Stereotyping and Internalization of the Thin Ideal in Preschool Girls," *Sex Roles* 63, no. 9 (2010): 615–616.

46 Phebe Cramer and Tiffany Steinwert, "Thin Is Good, Fat Is Bad: How Early Does It Begin?" *Journal of Applied Developmental Psychology* 19, no. 3 (1998): 429–451.

47 Carol K. Sigelman, Thomas E. Miller, and Laura A. Whitworth, "The Early Development of Stigmatizing Reactions to Physical Differences," *Journal of Applied Developmental Psychology* 7, no. 1 (1986): 17–32.

48 Cramer and Steinwert, "Thin Is Good."

49 Jane Wardle, Chloe Volz, and C. Golding, "Social Variation in Attitudes to Obesity in Children," *International Journal of Obesity* 19, no. 8 (1995): 562–569.

50 Marika Tiggemann and Elise Wilson-Barrett, "Children's Figure Ratings: Relationship to Self-Esteem and Negative Stereotyping," *International Journal of Eating Disorders* 23, no. 1 (1998): 83–88.

51 Dianne Neumark-Sztainer, Mary Story, and Loren Faibisch, "Perceived Stigmatization among Overweight African-American and Caucasian Adolescent Girls," *Journal of Adolescent Health* 23 (1998): 264–270.

52 Colleen S. W. Rand and Beatrice A. Wright, "Continuity and Change in the

Evaluation of Ideal and Acceptable Body Sizes across a Wide Age Span," *International Journal of Eating Disorders* 28, no. 1 (2000): 90–100; Janet D. Latner, Albert J. Stunkard, and G. Terence Wilson, "Stigmatized Students: Age, Sex, and Ethnicity Effects in the Stigmatization of Obesity," *Obesity Research* 13, no. 7 (2005): 1226–1231.

53 Linda Smolak and Michael P. Levine, "A Two-Year Follow-Up of a Primary Prevention Program for Negative Body Image and Unhealthy Weight Regulation," *Eating Disorders* 9, no. 4 (2001): 313–325.

54 Jacinta Lowes and Marika Tiggemann, "Body Dissatisfaction, Dieting Awareness and the Impact of Parental Influence in Young Children," *British Journal of Health Psychology* 8, no. 2 (2003): 135–147.

55 Elizabeth Goodman and Robert C. Whitaker, "A Prospective Study of the Role of Depression in the Development and Persistence of Adolescent Obesity," *Pediatrics* 110, no. 3 (2002): 497–504; Latner, Stunkard, and Wilson, "Stigmatized Students"; Puhl and Brownell, "Psychosocial Origins of Obesity Stigma"; Diane M. Quinn and Jennifer Crocker, "When Ideology Hurts: Effects of Belief in the Protestant Ethic and Feeling Overweight on the Psychological Well-Being of Women," *Journal of Personality and Social Psychology* 77, no. 2 (1999): 402–414; Marlene B. Schwartz, Lenny R. Vartanian, Brian A. Nosek, and Kelly D. Brownell, "The Influence of One's Own Body Weight on Implicit and Explicit Anti-Fat Bias," *Obesity* 14, no. 3 (2006): 440–447; Shirley S. Wang, Kelly D. Brownell, and Thomas A. Wadden, "The Influence of the Stigma of Obesity on Overweight Individuals," *International Journal of Obesity* 28, no. 10 (2004): 1333–1337.

56 Katherine A. Kraig and Pamela K. Keel, "Weight-Based Stigmatization in Children," *International Journal of Obesity* 25 (2001): 1661–166; Marika Tiggemann and Tracy Anesbury, "Negative Stereotyping of Obesity in Children: The Role of Controllability Beliefs," *Journal of Applied Social Psychology* 30, no. 9 (2000): 1977–1993.

57 Rebecca M. Puhl and Janet D. Latner, "Stigma, Obesity, and the Health of the Nation's Children"; Zeller and Modi, "Predictors of Health-Related Quality of Life in Obese Youth"; Dianne Neumark-Sztainer, Nicole Falkner, Mary Story, Cheryl Perry, Peter. J. Hannan, and Scott Mulert, "Weight-Teasing amongst Adolescents: Correlations with Weight Status and Disordered Eating Behaviours," *International Journal of Obesity* 26 (2002): 123–131.

58 Richard S. Strauss and Harold A. Pollack, "Social Marginalization of Overweight Children," *Archives of Pediatrics & Adolescent Medicine* 157, no. 8 (2003): 746–752.

59 Mir M. Ali, Aliaksandr Amialchuk, and John A. Rizzo, "The Influence of Body Weight on Social Network Ties among Adolescents," *Economics & Human Biology* 10, no. 1 (2012): 20–34.

60 Nicole H. Falkner, Dianne Neumark-Sztainer, Mary Story, Robert W. Jeffery, Trish Beuhring, and Michael D. Resnick, "Social, Educational, and Psychological Correlates of Weight Status in Adolescents," *Obesity Research* 9, no. 1 (2001): 32–42. After controlling for grade level, race, and socioeconomic status (SES), obese girls were less likely to interact with friends than were nonobese peers, and obese boys were less likely to spend time with friends and more likely to report that they felt their friends did not care about them than were nonobese boys.

61 Puhl and Latner, "Stigma, Obesity, and the Health of the Nation's Children," 557–580.

62 Neumark-Sztainer et al., "Weight Teasing."
63 Kelly D. Brownell, Marlene B. Schwartz, Rebecca M. Puhl, Kathryn E. Henderson, and Jennifer L. Harris, "The Need for Bold Action to Prevent Adolescent Obesity," *Journal of Adolescent Health* 45, no. 3 (2009): S8–S17.
64 Joanne Williams, Melissa Wake, Kylie Hesketh, Elise Maher, and Elizabeth Waters, "Health-Related Quality of Life of Overweight and Obese Children," *JAMA* 293, no. 1 (2005): 70–76; Margaret H. Zeller and Avani C. Modi, "Predictors of Health-Related Quality of Life in Obese Youth," *Obesity* 14, no. 1 (2006): 122–130.
65 Jeffrey B. Schwimmer, Tasha M. Burwinkle, and James W. Varni, "Health-Related Quality of Life of Severely Obese Children and Adolescents," *JAMA* 289 (2003): 1813–1819.
66 Ashlesha Datar and Roland Sturm, "Childhood Overweight and Elementary School Outcomes," *International Journal of Obesity* 30 (2006): 1449–1460.
67 Robert Crosnoe and Chandra Muller, "Body Mass Index, Academic Achievement, and School Context: Examining the Educational Experiences of Adolescents at Risk of Obesity," *Journal of Health and Social Behavior* 45, no. 4 (2004): 393–407.
68 Robert Crosnoe, "Gender, Obesity, and Education," *Sociology of Education* 80 (2007): 241–260. Crosnoe found that, following high school graduation, obese adolescent girls were less likely to attend college and had higher levels of self-rejection, class failure, and truancy than their nonobese peers.
69 Christian S. Crandall, "Do Parents Discriminate against Their Heavyweight Daughters?" *Journal of Personality and Social Psychology* 21, no.7 (1995): 724–737.
70 Michael J. Merten, K. A. S. Wickrama, and Amanda L. Williams, "Adolescent Obesity and Young Adult Psychosocial Outcomes: Gender and Racial Differences," *Journal of Youth and Adolescence* 37, no. 9 (2008): 1111–1122.
71 Xiaojia Ge, Glen H. Elder Jr., Mark Regnerus, and Christine Cox, "Pubertal Transitions, Perceptions of Being Overweight, and Adolescents' Psychological Maladjustment: Gender and Ethnic Differences," *Social Psychology Quarterly* 64, no. 4 (2001): 363–375. Ge et al. found that pubertal development and its associated weight gains were significantly linked to perceptions of being overweight—particularly among girls—and that these perceptions increase the risk of depressed moods, somatic complaints, and lower self-esteem among both genders. Belinda L. Needham and Robert Crosnoe, "Overweight Status and Depressive Symptoms during Adolescence," *Journal of Adolescent Health* 36, no. 1 (2005): 48–55.
72 Rebecca M. Puhl and Janet D. Latner, "Stigma, Obesity, and the Health of the Nation's Children," *Psychological Bulletin* 133, no. 4 (2007): 557–580.
73 Erving Goffman, *Stigma: Notes on the Management of a Spoiled Identity* (Englewood Cliffs, NJ: Prentice Hall, 1963).
74 Ellen M. Granberg, "Now My 'Old Self' Is Thin": Stigma Exits after Weight Loss," *Social Psychology Quarterly* 74, no. 1 (2011): 29–52.
75 Laura Backstrom, "From the Freak Show to the Living Room: Cultural Representations of Dwarfism and Obesity," *Sociological Forum* 27, no. 3 (2012): 682–707.
76 "100 Million Dieters, $20 Billion: The Weight-Loss Industry by the Numbers," *ABC News,* May 8, 2012. https://abcnews.go.com/Health/100-million-dieters-20-billion-weight-loss-industry/story?id=16297197.
77 Lee F. Monaghan, *Men and the War on Obesity: A Sociological Study* (London: Routledge, 2008).
78 Abigail C. Saguy and Anna Ward, "Coming Out as Fat: Rethinking Stigma," *Social Psychology Quarterly* 74, no. 1 (2011): 53–75.

79 Abigail C. Saguy, *What's Wrong with Fat?* (Oxford: Oxford University Press, 2013).
80 Saguy, *What's Wrong with Fat?*, 173.
81 Saguy, *What's Wrong with Fat?*
82 Sandra Lee Bartky, "Foucault, Femininity, and the Modernization of Patriarchal Power," in *Feminist Social Thought*, ed. Diana Tiegjens Meyer, 93–111 (New York: Routledge, 1997). Susan Bordo, *Unbearable Weight: Feminism, Western Culture, and the Body* (Berkeley: University of California Press, 1993): 93–111; Kandi M. Stinson, *Women and Dieting Culture: Inside a Commercial Weight Loss Group* (New Brunswick, NJ: Rutgers University Press, 2001); Cressida J. Heyes, "Foucault Goes to Weight Watchers," *Hypatia* 21, no. 2 (2006): 126–149.
83 Debra Gimlin, *Body Work: Beauty and Self-Image in American Culture* (University of California Press, 2001).
84 Natalie Allon, "Latent Social Services in Group Dieting," *Social Problems* 23, no. 1 (1975): 59–69.
85 Daniel D. Martin, "Organizational Approaches to Shame: Avowal, Management, and Contestation," *Sociological Quarterly* 41, no. 1 (2000): 125–150.
86 Stinson, *Women and Dieting Culture.*
87 Ellin, *Teenage Waistland.*
88 "My Week at the Biggest Loser Fat Camp," *New York Times*, January 1, 2012, TR1.
89 Ellin, *Teenage Waistland.*
90 "Priced Out of Weight Loss Camp," *New York Times*, August 8, 2016, C1.
91 Kristina P. Kelly and Dan S. Kirschenbaum, "Immersion Treatment of Childhood and Adolescent Obesity: The First Review of a Promising Intervention." *Obesity Reviews* 12, no. 1 (2011): 37–49.
92 Paul J. Gately, Carlton B. Cooke, Julian H. Barth, Bridgette M. Bewick, Duncan Radley, and Andrew J. Hill, "Children's Residential Weight-Loss Programs Can Work: A Prospective Cohort Study of Short-Term Outcomes for Overweight and Obese Children," *Pediatrics* 116, no. 1 (2005): 73–77.
93 Kelly Walker Lowry, Bethany J. Sallinen, and David M. Janicke, "The Effects of Weight Management Programs on Self-Esteem in Pediatric Overweight Populations," *Journal of Pediatric Psychology* 32, no. 10 (2007): 1179–1195.

Chapter 2   Studying Camp Odyssey

1 Hanne Warming, "Getting under Their Skins? Accessing Young Children's Perspectives through Ethnographic Fieldwork." *Childhood* 18, no. 1 (2011): 139–153.
2 Theresa Wiseman, "A Concept Analysis of Empathy," *Journal of Advanced Nursing* 23, no. 6 (1996): 1162–1167.
3 Carol A. B. Warren, and Tracy X. Karner, *Discovering Qualitative Methods: Field Research, Interviews, and Analysis*, 2nd ed. (New York: Oxford University Press, 2010).
4 Wiseman, "A Concept Analysis of Empathy," 1165.
5 Cate Watson, "The 'Impossible' Vanity: Uses and Abuses of Empathy in Qualitative Inquiry." *Qualitative Research* 9, no. 1 (2009): 105–117.
6 Patti Lather, "Against Empathy, Voice and Authenticity" in *Voice in Qualitative Inquiry: Challenging Conventional, Interpretive, and Critical Conceptions in Qualitative Research*, ed. Alecia Youngblood Jackson and Lisa Mazzei, 17–26 (London, Routledge, 2009).

7   Kathleen Blee, "White-Knuckle Research: Emotional Dynamics in Fieldwork with Racist Activists," *Qualitative Sociology* 21, no. 4 (1998): 381–399.
8   Warren and Karner, *Discovering Qualitative Methods*, 101.
9   Erving Goffman, *The Presentation of Self in Everyday Life* (New York: Doubleday, 1959).
10 Jocelyn Elise Crowley, "Friend or Foe? Self-Expansion, Stigmatized Groups, and Researcher-Participant Relationship," *Journal of Contemporary Ethnography* 36, no. 6 (2007): 603–630.
11 Julie Bettie, *Women without Class: Girls, Race, and Identity* (Berkeley: University of California Press, 2003), 25–26.
12 William Corsaro, *"We're Friends, Right?" Inside Kids' Culture* (Washington, DC: Joseph Henry Press, 2003).
13 Nancy Mandell, "The Least-Adult Role in Studying Children," *Journal of Contemporary Ethnography* 16, no. 4 (1988): 433–467.
14 Patricia Adler and Peter Adler. *Peer Power: Preadolescent Culture and Identity* (New Brunswick, NJ: Rutgers University Press, 1998); Hilary Levey, "'Which One Is Yours?' Children and Ethnography," *Qualitative Sociology* 32, no. 3 (2009): 311–331; Michael Messner, "Barbie Girls versus Sea Monsters: Children Constructing Gender," *Gender and Society* 14, no. 6 (2000): 765–784.
15 Sharlene Hesse-Biber, "The Practice of Feminist In-Depth Interviewing," in *Feminist Research Practice: A Primer*, ed. S. Hesse-Biber and P. Leavy, 111–148 (London: Sage, 2007).
16 Robert M. Emerson, Rachel I. Fretz, and Linda L. Shaw, *Writing Ethnographic Fieldnotes* (Chicago: University of Chicago Press, 1995).
17 Charles Briggs, *Learning How to Ask: A Sociolinguistic Appraisal of the Role of the Interview in Social Science Research* (Cambridge: Cambridge University Press, 1986).

Chapter 3   Learning Embodied Inequality through Social Comparisons

1   Charles H. Cooley, *Human Nature and the Social Order* (New York: Scribner, 1922 [1964]).
2   George H. Mead, *Mind, Self, and Society* (Chicago: University of Chicago Press, 1934).
3   Leon Festinger, "A Theory of Social Comparison Processes," *Human Relations* 7, no. 2 (1954): 117–140.
4   Diane Carlson Jones, "Social Comparison and Body Image: Attractiveness Comparisons to Models and Peers among Adolescent Girls and Boys," *Sex Roles* 45, no. 9/10 (2001): 645–664.
5   Donna Eder, Catherine Colleen Evans, and Stephen Parker, *School Talk: Gender and Adolescent Culture* (New Brunswick, NJ: Rutgers University Press, 1995); Melissa A. Milkie, "Social Comparisons, Reflected Appraisals, and Mass Media: The Impact of Pervasive Beauty Images on Black and White Girls' Self-Concepts," *Social Psychology Quarterly* 62, no. 2 (1999): 190–210; Mimi Nichter, *Fat Talk: What Girls and Their Parents Say about Dieting* (Cambridge, MA: Harvard University Press, 2000); Susan J. Paxton., Melinda Norris, Eleanor H. Wertheim, Sarah J. Durkin, and Jenny Anderson, "Body Dissatisfaction, Dating, and Importance of Thinness to Attractiveness in Adolescent Girls," *Sex Roles* 53, no. 9/10 (2005), 663–675.

6   Marika Tiggemann, "Body Dissatisfaction and Adolescent Self-Esteem: Prospective Findings," *Body Image* 2, no. 2 (2005): 129–135.

7   Cecilia L. Ridgeway, *Framed by Gender: How Gender Inequality Persists in the Modern World* (New York: Oxford University Press, 2011); Sauder, Michael, "Symbols and Contexts: An Interactionist Approach to the Study of Social Status," *Sociological Quarterly* 46, no. 2 (2005): 279–298.

8   Eder, Evans, and Parker, *School Talk*.

9   Timothy J. Halliday and Sally Kwak, "Weight Gain in Adolescents and Their Peers," *Economics and Human Biology* 7 no. 2 (2009): 181–190.

10 Murray Milner Jr., *Freaks, Geeks, and Cool Kids: Teenagers in an Era of Consumerism, Standardized Tests, and Social Media* (New York: Routledge, 2016).

11 Julie Guthman, *Weighing In: Obesity, Food Justice, and the Limits of Capitalism* (Berkeley: University of California Press, 2011).

12 Sandra Lee Bartky, "Foucault, Femininity, and the Modernization of Patriarchal Power," in *Feminist Social Thought*, ed. Diana Tiegjens Meyer, 93–111 (New York: Routledge, 1997).

13 Lynn Phillips, *Flirting with Danger: Young Women's Reflections on Sexuality and Domination* (New York: NYU Press, 2000), 40.

14 Hesse-Biber, *The Cult of Thinness*.

15 Cecelia Hartley, "Letting Ourselves Go: Making Room for the Fat Body in Feminist Scholarship," in *Bodies Out of Bounds: Fatness and Transgression*, ed. J. E. Braziel and K. LeBesco, 63 (Berkeley: University of California Press, 2001).

16 Natalie Boero, *Killer Fat: Media, Medicine, and Morals in the American "Obesity Epidemic"* (New Brunswick, NJ: Rutgers University Press, 2012). Boero also finds that this is the case for weight-loss surgery participants who reward themselves with shopping rather than food.

17 Xiaojia Ge, Glen H. Elder Jr., Mark Regnerus, and Christine Cox, "Pubertal Transitions, Perceptions of Being Overweight, and Adolescents' Psychological Maladjustment: Gender and Ethnic Differences," *Social Psychology Quarterly* 64, no. 4 (2001): 363–375; Michelle J. Pearce, Julie Boergers, and Mitchell J. Prinstein, "Adolescent Obesity, Overt and Relational Peer Victimization, and Romantic Relationships," *Obesity Research* 10 (2002): 386–393.

18 Jeanett L. Tang-Péronard, and Berit L. Heitmann, "Stigmatization of Obesity, The Importance of Gender," *Obesity Reviews* 9 (2008): 522–534.

19 Jeannine Gailey, *The Hyper(in)visible Fat Woman: Weight and Gender Discourse in Contemporary Society* (New York: Palgrave Macmillan, 2014).

20 Brent Harger, "You Say Bully, I Say Bullied: School Culture and Definitions of Bullying in Two Elementary Schools," in *Sociological Studies of Children and Youth, Volume 20*, ed. Y. Besen-Cassino, 95–123 (Bingley, U.K.: Emerald, 2016).

21 Mary B. Harris, "Is Love Seen as Different for the Obese?" *Journal of Applied Social Psychology* 20, no.15 (1990): 1209–1224.

22 Pearce, Boergers, and Prinstein, "Adolescent Obesity, Overt and Relational Peer Victimization."

23 Ibid.

24 Mark V. Roehling, Patricia Roehling, and Shaun Pichler, "The Relationship between Body Weight and Perceived Weight Related Discrimination: The Role of Sex and Race," *Journal of Vocational Behavior* 71, no. 2 (2007): 300–318.

25 Paxton et al., "Body Dissatisfaction"; Mary Lynn Damhorst, John M. Littrell, and

Mary Ann Littrell, "Age Differences in Adolescent Body Satisfaction," *Journal of Psychology* 121, no. 6 (1987): 553–562.
26 Sarah Mustillo, Kimber L. Hendrix, and Markus H. Schafer, "Trajectories of Body Mass and Self-Concept in Black and White Girls: The Lingering Effects of Stigma," *Journal of Health and Social Behavior* 53, no. 1 (2012): 2–16; Ellen M. Granberg, "Now My 'Old Self' Is Thin": Stigma Exits after Weight Loss," *Social Psychology Quarterly* 74, no. 1 (2011): 29–52.

Chapter 5   "They Were Born Lucky"

1 Kathleen S. Crittenden, "Sociological Aspects of Attribution," *Annual Review of Sociology* 9 (1983): 425–446.
2 Bernard Weiner, "Achievement Motivation as Conceptualized by an Attribution Theorist," in *Achievement Motivation and Attribution Theory*, ed. Bernard Weiner, 3–48 (Morristown, NJ: General Learning Press, 1974); Bernard Weiner, "The Development of an Attribution-Based Theory of Motivation: A History of Ideas," *Educational Psychologist* 45, no. 1 (2010): 28–36.
3 Kandi M. Stinson, *Women and Dieting Culture: Inside a Commercial Weight Loss Group* (New Brunswick, NJ: Rutgers University Press, 2001).

Chapter 6   Change Your Body, Change Yourself

1 Allison T. Chappell and Lonn Lanza-Kaduce, "Police Academy Socialization: Understanding the Lessons Learned in a Paramilitary-Bureaucratic Organization," *Journal of Contemporary Ethnography* 39, no. 2 (2010): 187–214; Renee C. Fox," The Autopsy: It's Place in the Attitude-Learning of Second-Year Medical Students," in *Essays in Medical Sociology: Journeys into the Field*, ed. Renée Fox, 51–77 (New Brunswick, NJ: Transaction Publishers, 1988); Robert K. Merton, George G. Reader, and Patricia L. Kendall, *The Student-Physician: Introductory Studies in the Sociology of Medical Education* (Cambridge, MA: Harvard University Press, 1957).
2 Erving Goffman, *Asylums: Essays on the Social Situations of Mental Patients and Other Inmates* (New York: Doubleday, 1961); Thomas Schmid and Richard Jones, "Suspended Identity: Identity Transformation in a Maximum Security Prison," *Symbolic Interaction* 14, no. 4 (1991): 415–432.
3 Jeylan T. Mortimer and Roberta G. Simmons, "Adult Socialization," *Annual Review of Sociology* 4 (1978): 421–454.
4 William Corsaro and Donna Eder, "Development and Socialization of Children and Adolescents," in *Sociological Perspectives on Social Psychology*, ed. Karen S. Cook, Gary Allan Fine, and James S. House, 421–451 (New York: Allyn and Bacon, 1995); Donna Eder and Sandi Kawecka Nenga, "Socialization in Adolescence," in *Handbook of Social Psychology*, ed. John Delamater, 157–182 (New York: Kluwer, 2003); Robin W. Simon, Donna Eder, and Cathy Evans, "The Development of Feeling Norms Underlying Romantic Love among Adolescent Females," *Social Psychology Quarterly* 55 (1992): 29–46.
5 Goffman, *Asylums*.
6 Chris Shilling, *The Body and Social Theory* (London: Sage, 2003), 4.
7 Centers for Disease Control and Prevention (CDC), "Vital Signs: State-Specific Obesity Prevalence Among Adults—United States, 2009," *Morbidity and*

Mortality Weekly Report 59 (2010), 1–5; Monica L. Baskin, Jamy D. Ard, Frank Franklin, and David Allison, "Prevalence of Obesity in the United States," *Obesity Reviews* 6, no. 1 (2005): 5–7; Qi Zhang and Youfa Wang, "Are American Children and Adolescents of Low Socioeconomic Status at Increased Risk of Obesity?" *American Journal of Clinical Nutrition* 84, no. 4 (2006): 707–716; John J. Reilly, Julie Armstrong, Ahmad Dorosty, Pauline Emmett, A. Ness, I. Rogers, Colin Steer and Andrea Sheriff, "Early Life Risk Factors for Obesity in Childhood: Cohort Study," *British Medical Journal* 330 (2005): 1357; Nancy E. Adler and Judith Stewart, "Reducing Obesity: Motivating Action While Not Blaming the Victim," *Milbank Quarterly* 87, no. 1 (2009): 49–70; Julie Guthman, *Weighing In: Obesity, Food Justice, and the Limits of Capitalism* (Berkeley: University of California Press, 2011); Lisa M. Powell, Christopher M. Auld, Frank J. Chaloupka, Patrick O'Malley, and Lloyd D. Johnston, "Associations between Access to Food Stores and Adolescent Body Mass Index," *American Journal of Preventive Medicine* 33, no. 4 (2007): S301–S307; Julie Guthman and Melanie DuPuis, "Embodying Neoliberalism: Economy, Culture and the Politics of Fat," *Environment and Planning D: Society and Space* 24, no. 3 (2006): 427–448.

8 Kristina Elfhag and Stephan Rossner, "Who Succeeds in Maintaining Weight Loss? A Conceptual Review of Factors Associated with Weight Loss Maintenance and Weight Regain," *Obesity Reviews* 6, no. 6 (2004): 67–85.

9 Susan Bordo, *Unbearable Weight: Feminism, Western Culture, and the Body* (Berkeley: University of California Press, 1993).

10 Bordo, *Unbearable Weight*, 201.

11 Loic Wacquant, *Body and Soul: Notebooks of an Apprentice Boxer* (New York: Oxford University Press, 2004).

12 Linda Bacon, *Health at Every Size: The Surprising Truth about Your Weight* (Dallas: BenBella Books, 2008); Steven N. Blair and Tim S. Church, "The Fitness, Obesity, and Health Equation: Is Physical Activity the Common Denominator?" *JAMA* 292 (2004): 1232–1234.

13 Shilling, *Body and Social Theory*.

14 Charles Edgley and Dennis Brissett, "Health Nazis and the Cult of the Perfect Body: Some Polemic Observations," *Symbolic Interaction* 13, no. 2 (1990): 257–279; Robert Crawford, "Healthism and the Medicalization of Everyday Life," *International Journal of Health Services* 10, no. 3 (1980): 356–388.

15 Abigail C. Saguy and Kjerstin Gruys, "Morality and Health: News Media Constructions of Overweight and Eating Disorders," *Social Problems* 57, no. 2 (2010): 231–250; Abigail C. Saguy, Kjerstin Gruys, and Shanna Gong, "Social Problem Construction and National Context: News Reporting on 'Overweight' and 'Obesity' in the U.S. and France," *Social Problems* 57, no. 4 (2010): 586–610.

16 Kandi M. Stinson, *Women and Dieting Culture: Inside a Commercial Weight Loss Group* (New Brunswick, NJ: Rutgers University Press, 2001); Natalie Allon, "Latent Social Services in Group Dieting," *Social Problems* 23, no. 1 (1975): 59–69; Daniel D. Martin, "Organizational Approaches to Shame: Avowal, Management, and Contestation," *Sociological Quarterly* 41, no. 1 (2000): 125–150.

17 Paul Campos, *The Obesity Myth* (New York: Gotham Books, 2004).

Chapter 7   The Benefits of Weight Loss Camp . . . and the Dark Side

1 Mimi Nichter, *Fat Talk: What Girls and Their Parents Say about Dieting* (Cambridge, MA: Harvard University Press, 2000).
2 Rachel Hannah Salk and Renee Engeln-Maddox, "Fat Talk among College Women Is Both Contagious and Harmful," *Sex Roles* 66, no. 9–10 (2012): 636–645.
3 Amy Barwick, Doris Bazzini, Denise Martz, Courtney Rocheleau, and Lisa Curtin, "Testing the Norm to Fat Talk for Women of Varying Size: What's Weight Got to Do with It?" *Body Image* 9, no. 1 (2012): 176–179.
4 Salk and Engeln-Maddox, "Fat Talk."

Conclusion

1 Michael Gard and Jan Wright, *The Obesity Epidemic: Science, Morality, and Ideology* (New York: Routledge, 2005); Gina Kolata, *Rethinking Thin: The New Science of Weight Loss—and the Myths and Realities about Dieting* (New York: Farrar, Straus and Giroux, 2007).
2 Julie Guthman, *Weighing In: Obesity, Food Justice, and the Limits of Capitalism* (Berkeley: University of California Press, 2011).
3 Paul Campos, *The Obesity Myth* (New York: Gotham Books, 2004).

Index

About the Author

LAURA BACKSTROM is an assistant professor of sociology at Florida Atlantic University. As a microsociologist, her research examines the cultural meanings of bodies in social interaction and how children negotiate social problems in their everyday lives.